...ess to Anaesthetics
Primary FRCA
Pocket Book 1:
Pharmacology and Clinical
MCQs

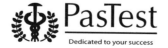

Dedicated to your success

Access to Anaesthetics Primary FRCA Pocket Book 1: Pharmacology and Clinical MCQs

Kirsty MacLennan MBChB, MRCP, FRCA

Specialist Registrar Anaesthesia

North West Region

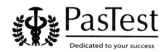

Dedicated to your success

© 2007 PASTEST LTD
Egerton Court
Parkgate Estate
Knutsford
Cheshire
WA16 8DX

Telephone: 01565 752000

First published 2007

ISBN: 1905 635 29X
ISBN: 978 1905 635 290

A catalogue record for this book is available from the British Library.

The information contained within this book was obtained by the author from
reliable sources. However, while every effort has been made to ensure its accuracy,
no responsibility for loss, damage or injury occasioned to any person acting or
refraining from action as a result of information contained herein can be accepted
by the publishers or author.

PasTest Revision Books and Intensive Courses

PasTest has been established in the field of postgraduate medical education since 1972, providing revision books and intensive study courses
for doctors preparing for their professional examinations.

Books and courses are available for the following specialties:
MRCGP, MRCP Parts 1 and 2, MRCPCH Parts 1 and 2, MRCPsych,
MRCS, MRCOG Parts 1 and 2, DRCOG, DCH, FRCA, PLAB Parts 1
and 2.

For further details contact:
PasTest, Freepost, Knutsford, Cheshire WA16 7BR
Tel: 01565 752000 Fax: 01565 650264
www.pastest.co.uk enquiries@pastest.co.uk

Typeset by Keytec Typesetting Ltd, Bridport, Dorset, UK
Printed and bound in the UK by Athenaeum Press, Gateshead

CONTENTS

ACKNOWLEDGEMENTS

I would like to thank Dr. Nolan for taking the time to write the foreword; Dr. Whitaker for his review; Dr. S. Maguire, Dr. K. Grady and Dr. W. de Mello for their advice and encouragement.

I would also like to thank the publishers, PasTest, my family, who have supported me. And above all, Ann MacLennan who has been my rock as always!

FOREWORD

The introduction of run-through training in Anaesthesia and the need for the Royal College of Anaesthetists [RCOA] to structure timing and content of Postgraduate examinations in accordance with the requirements of the Postgraduate Medical and Education Training Board [PMETB] has led to recent changes to the Primary Fellowship of the Royal College of Anaesthetists [FRCA] examination.

The Primary Multiple Choice Question [MCQ] examination became a "stand alone" Pass/Fail examination in June 2007. A close marking scheme is used where 1 is a poor fail, 1+ is a fail, 2 is a Pass and a 2+ reflects an outstanding performance. The Primary FRCA MCQ examination consists of 90 questions undertaken in three hours and comprises three subsections of 30 MCQs examining Pharmacology, Physiology, Physics and Clinical Measurement. A mark of 2 is required to pass the MCQ although a candidate who significantly underperforms in one or more subsection of the MCQ will fail the examination. Negative marking is applied with one mark being deducted for each incorrect answer.

A candidate may not proceed to the Objectively Structured Clinical Examination/Structured Oral Examination part of the Primary without passing the MCQ. An MCQ pass will be valid for a period of three years for a trainee working full time.

Although there is currently no limit on the number of attempts at this part of the examination, implicit in run through training is the need for trainees to achieve clinical competencies and examination milestones in a timely fashion.

It is generally acknowledged that an MCQ examination is a good test of core knowledge and there is no short cut to the acquisition of the considerable amount of information required to pass the Primary MCQ. Prospective candidates need to commit to an intensive programme of study of the syllabus supported by considerable practice of the technique of answering MCQs.

Dr Maclennan has produced a series of MCQs which cover in detail the Primary FRCA syllabus. The answer sections are clear and, where appropriate, supported by references to recent literature. Trainees commencing an anaesthesia training programme will find these MCQs useful to assess the depth of knowledge of the basic sciences which will be required of them, and those for whom the examination is imminent will find this series of books an invaluable means of self assessment and an indication of aspects of their knowledge and understanding which may need further work.

Dr D. Nolan, Regional Advisor for the North West

INTRODUCTION

Having taken both anaesthetic and medicine postgraduate examinations, I think that it is always difficult to know how best to start revising. It is important to avoid that unpleasant drowning sensation when you look at all the information that you have to absorb! I personally find that sitting and reading a textbook is time consuming, not particularly memorable and not especially useful for actually passing the exam. The best way to find out the gaps in your knowledge is to do as many practice MCQs as you can. This will stimulate you to read around the topics you are less familiar with, whilst improving your exam technique.

These books are different from others on the market as they are subject based. Many candidates feel that they have a particular area of weakness. These books will at worst highlight those weaknesses and at best, allow you to home in on specific topics, making them your areas of strength.

Each book contains 150 MCQs, covering pharmacology and clinical in book 1, physics, clinical measurement, equipment and statistics in book 2, physiology and anatomy in book 3. Within each book, the questions are mostly based in subject groups. This enables you to revise a particular topic or, you can always take a selection of questions from each book to make a practice exam paper.

The questions are based on the primary syllabus but will also be useful for candidates studying for the basic science part of the final examination.

Being pocket sized, there is now no excuse! Carry one in the pocket of your theatre blues and do a few questions before the patient arrives in the anaesthetic room or even over lunch!

The examination period is a stressful time, so make best use of *all* the time that you have.

Good luck!

Kirsty

Pharmacology

MCQs

Indicate your answers with a tick or cross in the boxes provided.

1.1 The following are true of cell membranes:

☐ A The lipophilic chains of the phospholipid bilayer of a cell membrane face outwards

☐ B Capillaries have fenestrae

☐ C Tight junctions exist in the blood–brain barrier, intestinal mucosa and renal tubules

☐ D Passive diffusion is the commonest method for substances to cross into a cell membrane

☐ E Ion channels may have their permeability changed by naturally occurring molecules or drugs

1.2 Regarding absorption of drugs:

☐ A The absorption of steroids across the gut lumen is an example of facilitated diffusion

☐ B Vitamin molecules are transported across the cell membrane via pinocytosis

☐ C The speed of absorption is predominantly dependent on lipid solubility

☐ D Lipid solubility affects the pharmacokinetics of absorption from a particular site

☐ E Severe hypoalbuminaemia will increase the amount of free basic drug available for absorption across a cell membrane

1.1   Answers:

- A False
- B True
- C True
- D True
- E True

Lipophilic chains face inwards.

Passive diffusion is the most common form of diffusion and requires no energy.

Ion channel permeability maybe altered according to other substances, for example local anaesthetic and fast-acting sodium channels.

1.2   Answers:

- A True
- B True
- C False
- D True
- E False

Pinocytosis is a mechanism of absorption. The cell membrane invaginates around the target molecule and moves it into the cell. It is a commonly utilised transport for large molecules.

The speed of absorption depends not only on lipid solubility but also on ionisation and protein binding.

α_1-Acid glycoprotein binds basic drugs whereas albumin tends to bind acidic or neutral drugs.

1.3 Ionisation:

☐ A The Henderson–Hasselbalch equation states:
$pH = pK_a + \log(\text{proton donor} \div \text{proton acceptor})$

☐ B For an acid (AH) the equation would read:
$pH = pK_a + \log([A^-] \div [AH])$

☐ C A base is more ionised in an environment that has a pH lower than its pK_a

☐ D The pK_a of blood at body temperature is 6.4

☐ E The pK_a is the pH at which 50% of the solution exists in ionised and unionised forms

1.4 Protein binding:

☐ A One albumin molecule can bind a number of different drugs

☐ B Albumin can bind to neutral drugs

☐ C Globins bind to basic drugs

☐ D Iron is bound to β_1-globin

☐ E Copper is bound to α_2-globin

1.3 Answers:

- A False
- B True
- C True
- D False
- E True

The Henderson-Hasselbalch equation states:
pH = pK_a + log([proton acceptor] ÷ [proton donor]).

Therefore, for a base (B), the equation would read:
pH = pK_a + log([B] ÷ [BH$^+$]).

The pK_a of blood at body temperature is 6.1.

1.4 Answers:

- A True
- B True
- C True
- D True
- E True

Albumin binds both neutral and acidic drugs whereas globins bind basic drugs. There are a number of different binding sites on an albumin molecule. Binding of one site can cause a conformational change and can alter ability to bind at other sites.

1.5 The acetylcholine receptor:

☐ A Is made up of five subunits in an adult: $\alpha \, \alpha \, \beta \, \delta \, \epsilon$

☐ B Requires the binding of two acetylcholine molecules in order to open the ion channel

☐ C Once open allows ions to pass at a rate of 10^7 per second

☐ D Demonstrates selectivity for the passage of sodium ions

☐ E Is activated following the arrival of an action potential as approximately 200 000 molecules of acetylcholine are released

1.6 Regarding cholinergic receptors:

☐ A They can be divided into nicotinic and muscarinic receptors

☐ B Muscarinic receptors are present on the postsynaptic membrane of neuromuscular junctions

☐ C Sweat glands contain muscarinic receptors

☐ D Salivary glands contain muscarinic receptors

☐ E They do not form a functioning part of the sympathetic nervous system

Pharmacology MCQs

1.5   Answers:

- A True
- B True
- C True
- D False
- E False

The acetylcholine receptor demonstrates selectivity for the passage of small cations but is not specific for sodium. It allows the passage of sodium, potassium and calcium across the membrane.

Approximately 2 million acetylcholine molecules are released per action potential.

Approximately 200 vesicles, each containing around 10 000 molecules of acetylcholine, are released per action potential.

1.6   Answers:

- A True
- B False
- C True
- D True
- E False

Nicotinic receptors are present in somatic muscle and at the ganglia of parasympathetic and sympathetic nerves, including sweat glands. They are also responsible for stimulation of the adrenal medulla.

Muscarinic receptors are found in the postganglionic parasympathetic nerve endings and in the postganglionic sympathetic nerve endings of the sweat glands. Postganglionic parasympathetic fibres supply the parotid, maxillary and sublingual salivary glands via muscarinic receptors.

Most postganglionic sympathetic effector function is via adrenergic receptors.

References: Yentis SM. *Anaesthesia and Intensive Care A–Z.* 3rd edn. Butterwoth Heinemann, 2004.
Power and Kam. *Principles of Physiology for the Anaesthetist.*

1.7   The following are true of neuromuscular blockade assessment:

- ☐ A Train of four (TOF) requires the application of a supramaximal stimulus at a frequency of 2 Hz
- ☐ B One twitch on a TOF is equivalent to 80% neuromuscular blockade
- ☐ C Seventy percent neuromuscular blockade is equivalent to three twitches on a TOF
- ☐ D Post-tetanic count is demonstrated by application of a 50-Hz stimulus for 5 seconds followed by a 3-second pause and then application of 2-Hz stimuli until the twitches disappear
- ☐ E Testing of neuromuscular blockade by use of orbicularis oculi can underestimate the degree of neuromuscular blockade

1.8   Suxamethonium:

- ☐ A Is chemically composed of two adjoined acetylcholine molecules
- ☐ B Has a longer duration of action compared with acetylcholine because its hydrolysing enzyme is not present at the neuromuscular junction
- ☐ C At approximately 50% of an administered dose reaches the neuromuscular junction
- ☐ D Is entirely hydrolysed in the plasma
- ☐ E At approximately 30% is excreted unchanged in the urine

1.7   Answers:

- A True
- B False
- C True
- D False
- E True

The TOF is a sequence of four supramaximal square wave electrical pulses each lasting 0.2 ms given at 2 Hz.

No twitch on a TOF corresponds to 100% blockade.

One twitch corresponds to 90% blockade.

Two twitches correspond to 80% blockade.

Three twitches correspond to 75% blockade.

Post-tetanic count is useful if there are no palpable/visible twitches on a TOF. A 5-second, 50-Hz tetanic stimulus is applied followed by a 3-second pause and then pulse stimulation at 1 Hz. The post-tetanic count is recorded. A count of 15 twitches is equivalent to 2 twitches on a TOF.

The orbicularis oculi muscle is less sensitive to neuromuscular blockade when compared with the diaphragm and vocal folds. The ulnar nerve is more sensitive.

1.8   Answers:

- A True
- B True
- C False
- D False
- E False

Introduced in the 1950s, suxamethonium offered significant advantages over the longer-acting tubocurarine used at the time. It is metabolised by plasma or pseudocholinesterases that are present in both plasma and liver, therefore very little of an administered dose actually reaches the neuromuscular junction (10–20%). It can exhibit phase 2 block, thought to be secondary to presynaptic blockade. Very little is excreted in the urine – approximately 10%.

Chemically it is two acetylcholine molecules, adjoined via their acetyl groups.

1.9   Suxamethonium:

☐ A Is metabolised to succinic acid and choline

☐ B Can cause nodal bradycardia secondary to sympathetic ablation

☐ C Can cause myalgia, which is most common in young women

☐ D Can cause a rise in intraocular pressure by approximately 100% for a matter of minutes after administration

☐ E Does not cause an increased risk of reflux as it increases the tone of the lower oesophageal sphincter

1.9   Answers:

- A True
- B False
- C True
- D True
- E True

Suxamethonium is initially metabolised to succinyl monocholine and then further metabolised to succinic acid and choline.

It can cause nodal bradycardia secondary to direct nodal muscarinic receptor stimulation.

Normal intraocular pressure (10–15 mmHg) is raised by ~100% following suxamethonium administration, which clearly presents a problem with penetrating eye injuries. Although it increases intragastric pressure by approximately 10 cmH_2O it also increases lower oesophageal sphincter tone and therefore does not increase the risk of reflux.

1.10   Regarding malignant hyperthermia:

☐   A   It exhibits autosomal recessive inheritance

☐   B   With increasing age there is a reduction in tendency to suffer a
             reaction

☐   C   It is associated with a defect on the receptor coded for on
             chromosome 19

☐   D   Without dantrolene mortality can approach 70%

☐   E   When anaesthetising a susceptible patient, the anaesthetic
             machine should first be flushed with 100% oxygen for 20–30
             minutes

1.10   Answers:

- A False
- B True
- C True
- D True
- E True

Malignant hyperthermia (MH) was thought to exhibit autosomal dominant inheritance; however, it now seems to be more complex than that and suspected cases should have DNA testing to reduce the risk of erroneous diagnosis.

It has been estimated that the UK population prevalence of genetic susceptibility lies between 1 : 5000 and 1 : 10 000.

It is associated with a defect on the ryanodine receptor, which is encoded for on chromosome 19, and results in an increase in intracellular calcium.

There seems to be a reduction in the tendency to have a reaction with increasing age. Interestingly, most patients found to be susceptible to MH will have had, on average, three previous uneventful anaesthetics.

With the introduction of dantrolene mortality is less than 5%. Dantrolene prevents the release of calcium from sarcoplasmic reticulum in striated muscle. It is presented as an orange powder containing 20 mg dantrolene, 3 g mannitol and sodium hydroxide. It is made up with 60 ml water, which gives the solution a pH of 9.5.

Dosage is 0.1 mg/kg to a maximum of 10 mg/kg.

Reference: Malignant hyperthermia. *British Journal of Anaesthesia CEPD Reviews* 2003; 3(1): 5–9.

1.11   Regarding suxamethonium apnoea:

- ☐ A   It can be congenital or acquired
- ☐ B   99% of the population are homozygous for the normal gene
- ☐ C   The gene for plasma cholinesterase activity is located on chromosome 19
- ☐ D   The dibucaine number represents the percentage inhibition that dibucaine (an amide local anaesthetic) causes to the plasma cholinesterase
- ☐ E   The dibucaine number of a homozygous normal genotype would be 80

1.12   Suxamethonium metabolism:

- ☐ A   There are 10 different genotypes responsible for suxamethonium metabolism
- ☐ B   Four different alleles have been identified in relation to pseudo/plasma cholinesterase activity
- ☐ C   The homozygous fluoride-resistant allele conveys the longest duration of action of suxamethonium
- ☐ D   Thyrotoxicosis is a cause for acquired suxamethonium apnoea
- ☐ E   Metoclopramide can cause acquired suxamethonium apnoea

1.11 Answers:

- A True
- B False
- C False
- D True
- E True

The gene encoding cholinesterase activity is on chromosome 3. Chromosome 19 encodes the ryanodine receptor, which is responsible for the condition malignant hyperthermia.

A total of 96% of the population are homozygous for the normal gene. Dibucaine inhibits normal plasma cholinesterase to a greater degree then abnormal cholinesterase. The dibucaine number represents this percentage inhibition, eg dibucaine inhibits the abnormal homozygous atypical gene by only 20%, giving a dibucaine number of 20.

1.12 Answers:

- A True
- B True
- C False
- D True
- E True

Ten different genotypes can occur from four different alleles.

The alleles are silent, atypical, fluoride resistant and normal.

Most prolonged suxamethonium duration is seen with homozygous silent, homozygous atypical and heterozygous silent atypical types.

Pathological causes of acquired suxamethonium apnoea include heart failure, renal failure, liver failure, hyperthyroidism and cancer.

Physiological causes include pregnancy and drug-induced causes secondary to the drug acting as either a substrate or an inhibitor (metoclopramide) to plasma cholinesterase.

1.13   When using non-depolarising muscle relaxants:

- [ ] A Concomitant use of lithium shortens the duration of neuromuscular blockade
- [ ] B Mivacurium is long-acting benzylisoquinolinium
- [ ] C Pancuronium is bisquaternary in nature
- [ ] D Vecuronium differs from pancuronium by a single methyl group
- [ ] E Rocuronium has a low potency compared with other aminosteroid muscle relaxants

1.14   Pancuronium:

- [ ] A Is associated with an increase in heart rate secondary to its blockade of cardiac muscarinic receptors
- [ ] B Has metabolites that are excreted in bile
- [ ] C Is more than 50% plasma protein bound
- [ ] D Is predominantly excreted unchanged in the urine
- [ ] E Is used in doses of 0.1 mg/kg to facilitate intubation

1.13   Answers:

- A   False
- B   False
- C   True
- D   True
- E   True

Lithium prolongs the action of non-depolarising muscle relaxants because of its sodium channel blockade effect.

Mivacurium is a short-acting benzylisoquinolinium lasting approximately 20 minutes.

1.14   Answers:

- A   True
- B   True
- C   False
- D   True
- E   True

Pancuronium is a bisquaternary aminosteroid muscle relaxant. Its use is associated with an increase in heart rate secondary to cardiac muscarinic receptor blockade and, because of indirect sympathomimetic activity, causes inhibition of norepinephrine reuptake at post-ganglionic nerve endings. It is between 10% and 40% protein bound. Around 35% is metabolised in the liver by deacetylation. Unchanged drug is excreted in the urine.

1.15   Vecuronium:

☐   A   Is stored as freeze-dried powder containing mannitol and sodium hydroxide

☐   B   Has been associated with myopathy when used as an infusion

☐   C   Is more lipid soluble than pancuronium

☐   D   Has a metabolite, 3-hydroxyvecuronium, that has significant muscle relaxant properties

☐   E   Causes tachycardia

1.16   Atracurium:

☐   A   Has four chiral centres

☐   B   Undergoes Hofmann elimination, which accounts for 60% of its metabolism

☐   C   Undergoes Hofmann elimination, which is increased by acidosis

☐   D   Yields laudanosine (a product of its metabolism), which is a glycine antagonist

☐   E   Yields laudanosine as a breakdown product of both Hofmann degradation and ester hydrolysis

1.15 Answers:

- A True
- B True
- C True
- D True
- E False

Vecuronium is a monoquaternary aminosteroid. It is unstable in solution and therefore is stored as a freeze-dried powder. It is more lipid soluble compared with pancuronium and has greater biliary excretion. Unlike pancuronium it is cardiac stable.

1.16 Answers:

- A True
- B False
- C False
- D True
- E True

Atracurium is a benzylisoquinolinium presented as a mixture of 10 stereoisomers. It has four chiral centres.

When used in intubating doses of 0.5 mg/kg it has a moderate duration of action.

Hofmann elimination accounts for 40% of its metabolism.

A total of 60% of it is metabolised by non-specific esterases.

Both elimination pathways yield laudanosine, a glycine antagonist, which has no neuromuscular blocking effects and is renally excreted.

1.17 **Regarding muscle relaxants:**

☐ A Cisatracurium is predominantly eliminated by Hofmann degradation

☐ B Cisatracurium is 10 times more potent than atracurium

☐ C Cisatracurium has active metabolites, ie with neuromuscular blocking properties

☐ D Cisatracurium is unsafe for use in patients with end-stage renal failure

☐ E Gallamine causes a tachycardia

1.18 **Edrophonium:**

☐ A Can worsen a cholinergic crisis

☐ B Forms a true covalent bond with acetylcholinesterase

☐ C Crosses the blood–brain barrier

☐ D Is predominantly excreted unchanged in the urine

☐ E Has a slower onset of action compared with neostigmine

1.17 Answers:

- A True
- B False
- C False
- D False
- E True

Cisatracurium, 1 of 10 stereoisomers present in atracurium, is three to four times more potent when compared with atracurium. It is predominantly excreted by Hofmann elimination, undergoing no direct plasma esterase hydrolysis. Metabolites are void of any neuromuscular blocking activity. It can be used safely in both renal and hepatic failure.

Gallamine, the first synthetic muscle relaxant, does cause increased heart rate secondary to cardiac muscarinic receptor blockade and sympathetic nervous system stimulation, like pancuronium.

1.18 Answers:

- A True
- B False
- C False
- D True
- E False

Edrophonium is used in the Tensilon test to aid diagnosis of myasthenia gravis. It inactivates acetylcholinesterase by forming weak electrostatic bonds with it, thereby blocking its active sites. It has a faster onset of action when compared with neostigmine and has fewer muscarinic side effects.

Edrophonium also causes an increase in acetylcholine release. It is a quaternary amine (like glycopyrrolate) and therefore does not cross the blood–brain barrier or the placenta.

Approximately 65% is excreted unchanged in urine with the remainder undergoing glucuronidation in the liver and bilious excretion.

1.19   Neostigmine:

☐ A   Forms a carbamylated enzyme complex with acetylcholinesterase

☐ B   May prolong the action of mivacurium

☐ C   Crosses the blood–brain barrier

☐ D   Is 50% excreted unchanged in the urine

☐ E   May precipitate bronchospasm in people with asthma

1.20   The following are true of anticholinesterase:

☐ A   Edrophonium may be a more appropriate reversal agent for mivacurium than neostigmine

☐ B   Physostigmine is well absorbed from the gut

☐ C   Organophosphorus compounds phosphorylate the anionic site of acetylcholinesterase, rendering it useless

☐ D   Acetylcholinesterase inhibitors can be used in the treatment of Alzheimer's disease

☐ E   Organophosphorus compounds can be used to treat narrow-angle glaucoma

1.19   Answers:

- A   True
- B   True
- C   False
- D   True
- E   True

Neostigmine is used as a reversal of neuromuscular blockade secondary to its action on acetylcholinesterase. It forms a carbamylated enzyme complex with acetylcholinesterase, thereby preventing the hydrolysis of acetylcholine.

Neostigmine is a quaternary compound and therefore does not cross the blood–brain barrier. It also inhibits plasma cholinesterase and can therefore lengthen the block of suxamethonium and mivacurium.

1.20   Answers:

- A   True
- B   True
- C   False
- D   True
- E   True

Mivacurium is metabolised by plasma cholinesterase, which neostigmine inhibits. Edrophonium, which increases acetylcholine release and decreases acetylcholine hydrolysis, would therefore be a more suitable aid to neuromuscular blockade reversal.

Physostigmine is a tertiary amine and therefore crosses the blood–brain barrier and placenta. Organophosphorus compounds irreversibly phosphorylate esteratic sites, rendering acetylcholinesterase useless.

Aricept (donepezil) is a reversible inhibitor of acetylcholinesterase, used in a once daily dose for the treatment of Alzheimer's disease. Ecothiopate is an example of an organophosphorus compound used for the treatment of narrow-angle glaucoma.

1.21   Regarding γ-aminobutyric acid (GABA) receptors:

☐ A GABA-A receptors are largely pre-synaptic

☐ B GABA-B receptors are ligand-gated ion channels

☐ C Activated GABA-B receptors increase chloride conductance

☐ D Benzodiazepines increase chloride conductance at the GABA-A receptor

☐ E Etomidate binds to the β subunit of GABA-A

1.22   Midazolam:

☐ A At pH < 3 it exists in an ionised form

☐ B Has a pK_a > 7.4

☐ C Causes pain on injection

☐ D Has effects that can be prolonged with concomitant administration of alfentanil

☐ E Has an oral bioavailability of approximately 70%

1.21   Answers:

- A   False
- B   False
- C   False
- D   True
- E   True

GABA-A receptors are ligand gated and largely postsynaptic. They potentiate chloride conductance.

GABA-B receptors are metabotropic, ie acting via G-proteins, and are associated with increased potassium conductance.

Both GABA-A and -B receptors cause hyperpolarisation of the neuronal membrane.

1.22   Answers:

- A   True
- B   False
- C   False
- D   True
- E   False

Midazolam is basic; when at pH 3.5 or less its ring structure is open and it exists as an ionised molecule. At pH > 3.5, its ring structure closes and it is unionised. Therefore, it exhibits tautomerism.

It has a pK_a of 6.5, ie at a pH 7.4 (plasma pH) it will exist predominantly in a unionised form (89% unionised) and is therefore lipid soluble. It is used as a water-soluble solution and it does not cause pain on injection.

Midazolam has an oral bioavailability of approximately 40%.

1.23   Regarding benzodiazepines:

☐   A   Diazepam is more highly protein bound than any of the other
        benzodiazepines

☐   B   Diazepam has a long elimination half-life compared with
        lorazepam

☐   C   Clearance of diazepam is greater than that of lorazepam

☐   D   Lorazepam has active metabolites

☐   E   Lorazepam has the highest volume of distribution

1.23   Answers:

- A False
- B True
- C False
- D False
- E False

Diazepam, lorazepam and midazolam are all approximately 95% protein bound.

Midazolam has the fastest elimination half-life followed by lorazepam then diazepam (1–4 hours, 10–20 hours and 20–45 hours, respectively).

The volume of distribution of diazepam and midazolam are approximately equal at 1–1.5 l/kg compared with 0.75–1.3 l/kg for lorazepam.

Clearance of midazolam is greater than that of lorazepam, which is greater than that of diazepam.

Diazepam and temazepam have active metabolites.

1.24   Tricyclic antidepressants:

☐ A Take effect as soon as the concentration of neurotransmitter in the synapse increases

☐ B Cause α-adrenoceptor blockade

☐ C Have a low volume of distribution

☐ D Are highly protein bound

☐ E In overdose may present with widening of the QRS complex on ECG

1.24   Answers:

- A False
- B True
- C False
- D True
- E True

The effect of tricyclic antidepressants does not mirror the increase in neurotransmitter at the synapse but occurs up to 2 weeks after administration.

Other effects include α-adrenoceptor, muscarinic and histaminergic blockade. They have a high volume of distribution and bind plasma proteins.

ECG changes include sinus tachycardia, ventricular arrhythmias, right bundle-branch block and prolonged QT.

Following overdose, most life-threatening problems occur within the first 6 hours. A greater risk of arrhythmias and seizures is observed with the following electrocardiograph (ECG) changes: widening of the QRS complex, increased QT interval and right axis deviation.

Reference: Cardiac arrest in special circumstances. *Advanced Life Support*. Resuscitation Council (UK). 5th edn. 122–3.

1.25   Regarding antidepressants:

☐ A Fluoxetine selectively blocks 5-HT neuronal reuptake

☐ B Venlafaxine blocks 5-HT and norepinephrine reuptake

☐ C Monoamine oxidase A preferentially deaminates tyramine and phenylethamine

☐ D Monoamine oxidase B preferentially deaminates 5-HT and catecholamines

☐ E New generation monoamine oxidase inhibitors are selective and reversible

1.26   Phenytoin:

☐ A Should be diluted with 5% dextrose

☐ B Inhibits cytochrome P450 enzymes

☐ C Initially undergoes zero-order kinetics

☐ D Has an oral bioavailability of approximately 50%

☐ E Has major metabolites that are excreted in bile

1.25   Answers:

- A True
- B True
- C False
- D False
- E True

Monoamine oxidase A deaminates 5-HT and catecholamines preferentially. Monoamine oxidase B deaminates tyramine and phenylethamine. New generation monoamine oxidase inhibitors, eg moclobemide, cause less potentiation of tyramine so the patients do not need dietary restrictions. Monoamine oxidase inhibitors have interactions that are important to anaesthesia. Indirectly acting sympathomimetics should be avoided, as these are reliant on monoamine oxidase for their metabolism. Directly acting sympathomimetics are also metabolised by catechol-*O*-methyltransferase and may therefore be used safely.

1.26   Answers:

- A False
- B False
- C False
- D False
- E False

Phenytoin is a widely used antiepileptic. It is also an anti-arrhythmic, neuroanalgesic and potent enzyme inducer. It inactivates sodium channels and may decrease calcium entry into neurons and enhance γ-aminobutyric acid (GABA) action. At low doses it undergoes first-order kinetics. Upon saturation of the enzyme system it undergoes zero-order metabolism. It has 90% oral bioavailability and major metabolites are excreted renally. Diluting with 5% dextrose is contraindicated as it is incompatible, becoming gelatinous.

1.27 The following are true of antacids:

☐ A The effects of sodium citrate wear off within 30 minutes

☐ B Cimetidine has an imidazole structure

☐ C Cimetidine is an H_1-receptor antagonist

☐ D Cimetidine is a hepatic microsomal enzyme inducer

☐ E Ranitidine is a hepatic microsomal enzyme inhibitor

1.28 Regarding antacids:

☐ A Ranitidine should be avoided in porphyria

☐ B Ranitidine can cause thrombocytopenia

☐ C Ranitidine has a high oral bioavailability

☐ D Famotidine is a proton pump inhibitor

☐ E Omeprazole achieves complete achlorhydria

1.27   Answers:

- A   True
- B   True
- C   False
- D   False
- E   False

Sodium citrate is a non-particulate antacid used extensively in obstetric anaesthesia. Cimetidine is an H_2-receptor antagonist. It increases gut pH and decreases volume of secretion. It is a cytochrome P450 enzyme inhibitor and 50% is excreted unchanged in urine. Ranitidine does not inhibit hepatic enzymes; however, it can cause reversible derangement of liver function tests (LFTs).

1.28   Answers:

- A   True
- B   True
- C   False
- D   False
- E   True

As with many drugs, ranitidine is not safe in porphyria. It may also cause thrombocytopenia and neutropenia, abnormal liver function tests (LFTs) and anaphylaxis. Oral bioavailability is 50%, as could be expected when comparing intravenous and oral drug dosages. Famotidine is a new H_2-receptor antagonist.

1.29   Drugs affecting the gastrointestinal tract:

☐ A Domperidone crosses the blood–brain barrier

☐ B Domperidone is readily available in intravenous preparations

☐ C Metoclopramide can cause acute hypertension in patients suffering with phaeochromocytoma

☐ D Cisapride has no antiemetic effect

☐ E High plasma levels of cisapride can precipitate serious arrhythmias, including torsades de pointes

1.30   Regarding local anaesthetics:

☐ A They are presented as hydrochloride salts

☐ B Their potency is attributed to ionisation

☐ C Their speed of action is attributed to lipid solubility

☐ D Their duration of action is attributed to protein binding

☐ E In general, local anaesthetics cause vasodilatation in high concentrations

1.29 Answers:

- A False
- B False
- C True
- D True
- E True

Domperidone does not cross the blood–brain barrier and as such is less likely to produce extrapyramidal side effects compared with metoclopramide. Domperidone (a dopamine antagonist) was previously given intravenously but was deemed unsafe secondary to serious arrhythmias, so now it is available only as oral or rectal preparations.

1.30 Answers:

- A True
- B False
- C False
- D True
- E False

Local anaesthetics are presented as hydrochloride salts, which leaves them water soluble. Potency is related to lipid solubility, speed of onset to pK_a (ie ionisation) and duration of action to protein binding. Low concentrations of local anaesthetics tend to cause vasodilatation whereas high concentrations tend to cause vasoconstriction.

1.31   Local anaesthetics:

- ☐ A   Dibucaine is an ester
- ☐ B   Systemic absorption is higher with a brachial plexus block compared with a caudal one
- ☐ C   Esters are less protein bound when compared with amides
- ☐ D   *p*-Aminobenzoate is an amide metabolite
- ☐ E   Esters do not cross the placenta in significant amounts

1.32   Pharmacological properties of amide local anaesthetics:

- ☐ A   The pK_a of bupivacaine is greater than the pK_a of procaine
- ☐ B   At physiological pH more than 40% of lidocaine is unionised
- ☐ C   Bupivacaine and ropivacaine have similar percentage protein binding
- ☐ D   Bupivacaine is more lipid soluble when compared with ropivacaine
- ☐ E   Amides are extensively protein bound to α1-acid glycoprotein

1.31   Answers:

- A   False
- B   False
- C   True
- D   False
- E   True

Dibucaine (used in the diagnosis of plasma cholinesterase deficiency) is an amide local anaesthetic. The highest systemic absorption is associated with intercostal blockade, then caudal, epidural and brachial plexus, and finally the lowest absorption with subcutaneous infiltration. *p*-Aminobenzoate is the main ester metabolite that infers its hypersensitivity trait. Esters are rapidly metabolised by plasma esterases so insignificant amounts cross the placenta.

1.32   Answers:

- A   False
- B   False
- C   True
- D   True
- E   True

The pK_a of bupivacaine is 8.1 compared with 8.9 for procaine. At physiological pH lidocaine is 25% unionised and 70% protein bound to α_1-acid glycoprotein. Both bupivacaine and ropivacaine are 95% protein bound. Amides are basic drugs and are therefore extensively bound to α_1-acid glycoprotein. Bupivacaine is approximately three times more lipid soluble when compared with ropivacaine.

1.33   Regarding commonly used topical local anaesthetics:

☐ A   EMLA (cream) is an oil at room temperature

☐ B   EMLA cream is a 50 : 50 mix of lidocaine and procaine

☐ C   EMLA must be allowed 60 minutes to work

☐ D   Amethocaine 4% cream applied topically has a duration of action of up to 6 hours

☐ E   Amethocaine should be avoided in patients with methaemoglobinaemia

1.34   Regarding local anaesthetics:

☐ A   Lidocaine exhibits class 1A anti-arrhythmic properties

☐ B   Only approximately 1% of an epidurally administered dose of bupivacaine crosses the placenta

☐ C   The *R* isomer of ropivacaine has less desirable pharmacological characteristics compared with the *S* isomer

☐ D   Cocaine is hepatically metabolised to inactive products

☐ E   Local anaesthetics are mixed with alkaline agents to increase their unionised fraction

1.33   Answers:

- A   True
- B   False
- C   True
- D   True
- E   False

EMLA is an example of a eutectic mixture. It is composed of a 50 : 50 mix of 2.5% lidocaine and 2.5% prilocaine. Prilocaine is metabolised to *O*-toluidine, which causes methaemoglobinaemia. EMLA cream requires 1 hour to provide effective analgesia, whereas amethocaine requires only 30 minutes and also produces vasodilatation, which aids with cannulation.

1.34   Answers:

- A   False
- B   True
- C   True
- D   True
- E   True

Lidocaine exhibits class 1B anti-arrhythmic properties that are used to treat ventricular arrhythmia. A total of 95% of a delivered dose of bupivacaine is protein bound and therefore unable to cross lipid membranes. Of the remaining 5% only 15% is unionised and therefore able to pass across the placenta, ie approximately 0.75% of delivered dose. Ropivacaine exists in two forms – *S* and *R* enantiomers. The *R* enantiomer is less potent and more toxic, so a pure *S* enantiomer form exists. As local anaesthetics are basic by increasing the pH, the drug exists more in its unionised form and is therefore able to cross nerve membranes.

1.35   The following agents are bacteriostatic rather than bactericidal:

☐ A Sulphonamides

☐ B Quinolones

☐ C Clindamycin

☐ D Co-trimoxazole

☐ E Macrolides

1.36   Regarding penicillins:

☐ A Phenoxymethylpenicillin (penicillin V) is unstable in acid conditions

☐ B Flucloxacillin is unaffected by β-lactamases

☐ C Clavulanic acid is an irreversible inhibitor of β-lactamases

☐ D Tazocin contains tazobactam (a β-lactamase inhibitor)

☐ E Aminoglycosides act synergistically with penicillins

1.35 Answers:

- A True
- B False
- C True
- D False
- E True

Bacteriostatic	Bactericidal
Macrolides	Penicillin
Tetracycline	Cephalosporins
Sulphonamide	Aminoglycosides
Chloramphenicol	Co-trimoxazole
Clindamycin	Isoniazid
Lincomycin	Vancomycin
	Metronidazole
	Quinolones

1.36 Answers:

- A False
- B True
- C True
- D True
- E True

Phenoxymethylpenicillin must be stable in acid as it is given as an oral preparation. Tazocin is a combination of piperacillin and tazobactam. Penicillins have their effect by binding transpeptidase, which is then unable to cross-link bacterial cell wall peptidoglycans.

1.37   Cephalosporins:

☐   A   Contain a β-lactam ring structure

☐   B   Of third-generation type (eg ceftriaxone) have a reduced
             Gram-negative action when compared with second-generation
             cephalosporins (eg cefuroxime)

☐   C   Undergo enhanced renal elimination with probenecid

☐   D   Are bactericidal

☐   E   Of second-generation type have good activity against *Neisseria
             gonorrhoeae*

1.38   The following are the correct methods of action of antibiotics:

☐   A   Tetracyclines inhibit bacterial protein synthesis by binding the
             50-S ribosome subunit

☐   B   Aminoglycosides inhibit bacterial protein synthesis by binding
             the 50-S ribosome subunit

☐   C   Ciprofloxacin inhibits transpeptidase action on peptidoglycans

☐   D   Metronidazole inhibits RNA gyrase

☐   E   Vancomycin binds transpeptidase, inhibiting cell wall
             synthesis

1.37   Answers:

- A True
- B False
- C False
- D True
- E True

Cephalosporins are also bacterial cell wall synthesis inhibitors.
Their β-lactam ring renders them less susceptible to β-lactamases
when compared with penicillins. There are three generations of
cephalosporins. The second generation is particularly effective
against *Haemophilus influenzae* and *Neisseria gonorrhoeae*. The
third generation has improved Gram-negative but less Gram-
positive cover when compared with second generation. As with
penicillins, probenecid prevents elimination by preventing its
renal secretion.

1.38   Answers:

- A False
- B False
- C False
- D False
- E False

Tetracyclines inhibit bacterial protein synthesis by binding to the
30-S ribosome and inhibiting tRNA. Macrolides bind to the 50-S
ribosome, inhibiting bacterial translocation. Ciprofloxacin (a
quinolone) is a DNA gyrase inhibitor. Metronidazole releases
agents that interfere with DNA synthesis and function.
Vancomycin acts in a similar way to penicillins by inhibiting cell
wall synthesis but inactivates the enzyme glycoprotein synthetase
not transpeptidase. Aminoglycosides cause misreading of mRNA
and bind to 30-S ribosomes, so inhibiting tRNA.

1.39   MAC (minimum alveolar concentration) of a volatile anaesthetic:

☐   A   Decreases with concurrent lithium administration

☐   B   Is a measure of potency

☐   C   Is increased in neonates

☐   D   Of isoflurane with nitrous oxide is approximately 0.8

☐   E   Of nitrous oxide is 105

1.40   Halothane:

☐   A   Has a molecular weight of 184

☐   B   Should not be administered concomitantly with drugs
            decreasing atrioventricular (AV) nodal conduction

☐   C   Can induce halothane hepatitis, with a greater incidence in
            children when compared with adults

☐   D   Is a safe alternative to sevoflurane when anaesthetising patients
            with head injury

☐   E   Has an oil : gas partition coefficient of 22.4

1.39 Answers:

- A True
- B True
- C False
- D True
- E True

There are a range of factors both increasing and decreasing MAC. Lithium administration, acute alcohol and opioid ingestion, neonatal period, hypometabolic states and concurrent nitrous oxide administration decrease MAC.

MAC is increased by hypermetabolic states, chronic alcohol and opioid use, and some metabolic derangements including hypernatraemia.

1.40 Answers:

- A False
- B True
- C False
- D False
- E False

Halothane has a molecular weight of 197, boiling point 50.2°C, MAC 0.75, blood : gas partition coefficient 2.4, oil : gas partition coefficient 224.

Adult incidence of halothane hepatitis is 1 in 2500–35 000 compared with that of 80 000–200 000 in children. Halothane significantly increases cerebral blood flow so increasing intracranial pressure and thereby decreasing cerebral perfusion pressure, which should be avoided in the head-injured patient. Halothane also causes an increased incidence of bradycardia secondary to its augmentation of vagal tone and sinoatrial (SA) and atrioventricular (AV) nodal depression, which can be exacerbated by concomitant medications.

1.41 The alveolar partial pressure of volatile agents increases more rapidly in patients with:

☐ A An increased functional residual capacity

☐ B Eisenmenger's syndrome

☐ C An increased cardiac output

☐ D Concomitant nitrous oxide administration

☐ E Fibrotic lung disease

1.42 Regarding volatile anaesthetics:

☐ A Isoflurane is presented as a racemic mixture

☐ B 0.2% of inhaled isoflurane is metabolised

☐ C Fluoride ion production secondary to enflurane metabolism is increased in obese patients

☐ D Abnormal electroencephalograph (EEG) activity is associated with high concentrations of enflurane in hypocapnic patients

☐ E At levels of 1 MAC of isoflurane, cerebral autoregulation is preserved

1.41 Answers:

- A False
- B True
- C False
- D True
- E True

An increase in functional residual capacity causes a greater dilution of the volatile agents, so decreasing alveolar partial pressure. A decreased functional residual capacity is associated with fibrotic lung disease and has the opposite effect, causing decrease in dilution and therefore increasing partial pressures. Eisenmenger's syndrome (a right-to-left intracardiac shunt) reduces the blood flow to the lungs and so increases the alveolar partial pressure of volatile agents. Nitrous oxide causes an increase in volatile partial pressures within the alveolar secondary to its second gas effect. An increased cardiac output improves the concentration gradient, promoting diffusion, and therefore reduces alveolar partial pressure.

1.42 Answers:

- A True
- B True
- C True
- D True
- E True

Isoflurane is the structural isomer of enflurane: 0.2% of isoflurane is metabolised compared with 2% of enflurane, <5% of sevoflurane and 0.02% of desflurane. Abnormal 3-Hz spike on an EEG is associated with high concentrations of enflurane in hypocapnic patients.

1.43   Sevoflurane:

- ☐ A   Is achiral
- ☐ B   Has a molecular weight of 200
- ☐ C   Has a saturated vapour pressure at 20°C of 22.7 kPa
- ☐ D   Decreases cerebral oxygen requirements
- ☐ E   Does not affect splanchnic blood flow

1.44   Regarding volatile anaesthetics:

- ☐ A   Desflurane has a boiling point of 21°C
- ☐ B   Desflurane is administered by a Tec 5 vaporiser
- ☐ C   Compound A has a molecular weight of 179
- ☐ D   More compound A is formed with baralyme compared with soda lime
- ☐ E   Xenon (^{133}Xe) may be used to measure cerebral blood flow

1.43   Answers:

- A True
- B True
- C True
- D True
- E True

The physiochemical properties of sevoflurane include a boiling point of 58.5°C, an MAC of 1.8%, blood : gas partition coefficient of 0.69 and an oil : gas partition coefficient of 80.

1.44   Answers:

- A False
- B False
- C True
- D True
- E True

Desflurane (boiling point 23.5°C) is administered in a Tec 6 vaporiser, which holds 450 ml and heats desflurane to 39°C at 2 atm. Compound A can be formed by reaction with both soda lime and baralyme. It is formed in increasing amounts with high temperatures. A greater temperature rise is seen with baralyme, therefore yielding greater amounts of compound A. The radioactive isotope ^{133}Xe may be used to determine cerebral and other organ blood flow.

1.45   Diuretics, thiazides:

☐   A   Exert their main hypotensive effects secondary to diuresis

☐   B   Cause hypokalaemia and hypochloraemic acidosis

☐   C   Increase bicarbonate excretion

☐   D   Increase plasma cholesterol level

☐   E   Can cause thrombocytopenia

1.46   The following are true of diuretics:

☐   A   Loop diuretics inhibit sodium and chloride reabsorption solely in the thick ascending limb of the loop of Henle

☐   B   Loop diuretics cause a decrease in renal blood flow

☐   C   Loop diuretics may cause a rise in lithium levels

☐   D   Canrenone is a metabolite of spironolactone

☐   E   Aldosterone antagonists are available in intravenous preparations

1.45   Answers:

- A False
- B False
- C True
- D True
- E True

Most diuretics, including thiazides and loop diuretics, exert their antihypertensive effect secondary to a decrease in systemic vascular resistance. Thiazides inhibit sodium and chloride reabsorption predominantly in the early distal convoluted tubule. The increase in sodium reaching the latter part of the distal tubule causes rapid sodium reabsorption in exchange for hydrogen and potassium ions. Therefore, the overall picture is that of hypokalaemia with hypochloraemic alkalosis

1.46   Answers:

- A False
- B False
- C True
- D True
- E True

Loop diuretics act mainly in the thick ascending limb of the loop of Henle, although they also have some action in the early distal tubule. Loop diuretics inhibit sodium and chloride reabsorption and increase renal blood flow (whereas thiazides decrease renal blood flow). An example of intravenous aldosterone antagonists is potassium canrenoate.

1.47 Diuretics:

- ☐ A Mannitol is a polyhydric alcohol
- ☐ B Mannitol may be harmful in head injury
- ☐ C Mannitol undergoes no significant metabolism
- ☐ D Acetazolamide competitively inhibits carbonic anhydrase
- ☐ E Acetazolamide renders urine alkaline

1.48 Sodium nitroprusside:

- ☐ A Is a prodrug
- ☐ B Causes inactivation of the enzyme guanylyl cyclase
- ☐ C Causes increased pulmonary shunt
- ☐ D Undergoes an initial metabolic reaction that yields methaemoglobin
- ☐ E Increases thiocyanate, which is then converted back to cyanide ion by the mitochondrial enzyme rhodanase

1.47   Answers:

- A True
- B True
- C True
- D False
- E True

Mannitol may be used in head injury to reduce oedema but must be used with care. If the blood–brain barrier is breached mannitol can enter into the brain tissue and draw fluid into it, so further increasing intracranial pressure. Acetazolamide (a carbonic anhydrase inhibitor) provides non-competitive blockade. It inhibits hydrogen ion and bicarbonate production from water and carbon dioxide. This causes a decrease in hydrogen excretion and decreased bicarbonate absorption, so leading to alkaline urine with a hyperchloraemic acidosis.

1.48   Answers:

- A True
- B False
- C True
- D True
- E False

Sodium nitroprusside is a prodrug. Nitric oxide is the active agent. This causes activation of guanylyl cyclase, causing venodilatation and arterial dilatation. It reduces pulmonary hypoxic vasoconstriction, so increasing pulmonary shunt. Its metabolism is complex. The initial metabolic pathway is within the red blood cell and following reaction with oxyhaemoglobin gives rise to nitric oxide, cyanide ions ($\times$ 5) and methaemoglobin. Methaemoglobin then combines with cyanide ions to form cyanomethaemoglobin. The remaining cyanide ions are converted to thiocyanate by the mitochondrial enzyme rhodanase. Other cyanide ions combine with vitamin B_{12} to form cyanocobalamin. Both thiocyanate and cyanocobalamin are renally excreted.

1.49   Regarding sodium nitroprusside metabolism:

☐ A Toxicity starts to occur as cyanide levels exceed 15 µg/ml

☐ B Cyanide toxicity is more common in the febrile patient

☐ C Sodium thiosulphate increases the production of cyanomethaemoglobin

☐ D Cyanide ion toxicity increases mixed venous oxygen saturation

☐ E Thiocyanate is not harmful

1.50   Regarding nitrates:

☐ A Induced hypotension is predominantly secondary to venodilatation

☐ B Tolerance is secondary to depletion of vascular smooth muscle sulphydryl groups

☐ C Isosorbide mononitrate has 100% oral bioavailability

☐ D The main effect of isosorbide dinitrate is conferred by its hepatic metabolites (isosorbide 2-mononitrate and isosorbide 5-mononitrate)

☐ E Nitrite release from nitrate metabolism oxidises the iron in oxyhaemoglobin

1.49   Answers:

- A False
- B False
- C False
- D True
- E False

Cyanide ion toxicity occurs at levels over 8 μg/ml and is more common in the hypothermic patient. Sodium thiosulphate increases conversion of cyanide ions to thiocyanate, most of which is excreted in the urine, therefore decreasing circulating cyanide ions. Although not as harmful as cyanide ions, if allowed to accumulate thiocyanate is harmful and can interfere with thyroid function. Cyanide ion toxicity causes inactivation of cytochrome oxidase and therefore impairs oxygen utilisation, so increasing mixed venous oxygen saturation.

1.50   Answers:

- A True
- B True
- C True
- D True
- E True

The hypotensive effect of nitrates is predominantly secondary to relaxation of the venous circulation although the arterial smooth muscle tone is also affected (to a lesser extent).

Remember **OIL** and **RIG** – **O**xidation **I**s **L**oss of electrons and **R**eduction **I**s **G**ain of electrons. Nitrite converts oxyhaemoglobin to methaemoglobin by oxidation of ferrous Fe^{2+} to ferric Fe^{3+}, ie loss of electrons. Owing to its lack of first-pass hepatic metabolism, isosorbide mononitrate has an oral bioavailability of 100%.

1.51   Drugs affecting coagulation:

☐ A Aspirin acts by irreversible methylation of platelet cyclo-oxygenase

☐ B Dipyridamole inhibits adenosine uptake into platelets

☐ C Dextrans are produced by bacteria

☐ D Dextrans have no effect on the function of von Willebrand's factor

☐ E Dextrans can impair crossmatching

1.52   Unfractionated heparin:

☐ A Is basic

☐ B Increases the formation of antithrombin III–thrombin inactive complex by a 1000-fold

☐ C Inhibits factor Xa only at high concentrations

☐ D Can affect factor XIIa

☐ E Does not cross the blood–brain barrier

1.51   Answers:

- A False
- B True
- C True
- D False
- E True

Aspirin irreversibly acetylates cyclo-oxygenase, so causing a reduction in thromboxane production. At low doses the platelet cyclo-oxygenase is inhibited whereas the vessel wall cyclo-oxygenase is unaffected and still able to confer its useful properties of prostaglandin synthesis and dilatation.

Dipyridamole is a potent coronary artery vasodilator. It inhibits phosphodiesterase and phospholipase activity. This renders the platelets less prone to aggregation. Dextrans are polysaccharides produced by the bacterium *Leuconostoc mesenteroides*; their anticoagulant activity is secondary to decreased platelet adhesiveness and von Willebrand's factor inhibition. It also produces a protective coating over vessel linings and red cells, so aiding flow in the microcirculation. Dextran 70 is known to interfere with crossmatching secondary to rouleaux formation.

1.52   Answers:

- A False
- B True
- C False
- D True
- E True

Heparin is a large acidic molecule, which increases the formation of the inactive antithrombin III–thrombin complex by ~1000-fold. At low doses factor Xa can be affected. Factors XIIa, XIa and IXa can be affected at high doses. Due to its large size and charged nature, it crosses neither the blood–brain barrier nor the placenta.

1.53   Unfractionated heparin:
- ☐ A   Is bound to fibrinogen in plasma
- ☐ B   Metabolites are excreted hepatically
- ☐ C   Decreases plasma turbidity
- ☐ D   Does not affect platelets, even at high doses
- ☐ E   Induced thrombocytopenia is antibody mediated

1.54   When using low-molecular-weight heparins (LMWHs):
- ☐ A   Protamine administration fully reverses the effect
- ☐ B   They have an increased factor Xa-inhibiting effect compared with unfractionated heparin
- ☐ C   They have increased affinity for von Willebrand's factor when compared with unfractionated heparin
- ☐ D   Monitoring of anti-factor Xa levels is recommended
- ☐ E   They affect activated partial thrombin time (APTT) results

1.53 Answers:

- A True
- B False
- C True
- D False
- E True

Heparin is negatively charged. In plasma it binds antithrombin III (so having its effect), albumin, protease and fibrinogen. It is metabolised by hepatic heparinases and its metabolites are excreted in urine. At low doses it inhibits factor Xa. At high doses it effects platelet aggregation and factors XIIa, XIa and IXa. Plasma turbidity is decreased secondary to the reduction in triglyceride levels. Heparin-induced thrombocytopenia (HIT) is an antibody-mediated condition occurring in 3% of patients approximately 5–10 days after initiation of therapy. Platelets are bound and removed from circulation, rendering the patient thrombocytopenic.

1.54 Answers:

- A False
- B True
- C False
- D False
- E False

Protamine, which reverses heparin fully at doses of 1 mg/100 IU heparin, does not fully reverse the effects of LMWH although it is still advocated in bleeding. LMWH has an increased affinity for factor Xa (which confers its main effect) but decreased affinity for von Willebrand's factor. Monitoring anti-factor Xa levels is not recommended, as it does not predict the risk of bleeding and is not therefore helpful. APTT is unaltered.

1.55   Regarding anticoagulation:

☐ A Fondaparinux produces its antithrombotic effect through factor Xa inhibition

☐ B Patients on single daily dose LMWH should have their epidural catheters removed no sooner than 6 hours after the last dose

☐ C Subsequent LMWH dosing should occur a minimum of 2 hours after catheter removal in patients on single daily dose LMWH

☐ D Neuroaxial blockade is thought to be safe to perform if the INR (international normalised ratio) is < 1.5

☐ E Clopidogrel should ideally be stopped 7 days before epidural insertion

1.56   Protamine:

☐ A Is prepared from fish eggs

☐ B Is a mixture of basic low-molecular-weight proteins

☐ C Is used in some insulin preparations

☐ D In individual doses should not exceed 1000 mg

☐ E With previous vasectomy may predispose to allergic reaction

1.55   Answers:

- A   True
- B   False
- C   True
- D   True
- E   True

Patients on LMWH delivered as a single daily dose should have their first postoperative dose given at 6–8 hours with their second postoperative dose no earlier than 24 hours after surgery. An epidural catheter should be removed no earlier than 10–12 hours after the last dose of LMWH. Once the catheter has been removed the LMWH dose can be given no earlier than 2 hours later.

Reference: Anticoagulants and the perioperative period.
Continuing Education in Anaesthesia, Critical Care and Pain.
British Journal of Anaesthetics 2006; 6(4):

1.56   Answers:

- A   False
- B   True
- C   True
- D   False
- E   True

Protamine is prepared from fish (including salmon) sperm and ironically enough previous vasectomy predisposes to allergic reaction – as does chronic diabetes and allergy to fish! It is basic and as such binds to the acidic heparin, forming a stable inactive salt. It is present in some insulin preparations. The recommended maximum dose is 50 mg.

1.57   Warfarin:

- ☐ A Is acidic
- ☐ B Binds to α_1-acid glycoprotein preferentially
- ☐ C Inhibits the synthesis of factor II
- ☐ D Inhibits the synthesis of factor VIII
- ☐ E Prevents the oxidation of vitamin K

1.58   Warfarin:

- ☐ A Is more than 95% protein bound
- ☐ B Is teratogenic, particularly in the second trimester
- ☐ C Metabolites are predominantly excreted in urine
- ☐ D Effects are antagonised by erythromycin
- ☐ E Effects are potentiated by barbiturates

1.57   Answers:

- A True
- B False
- C True
- D False
- E True

Warfarin is an acid that preferentially binds albumin. It inhibits the synthesis of vitamin K-dependent clotting factors, ie factors II, VII, IX and X. To activate these clotting factors they undergo γ-carboxylation of their glutamic acid residues; for this to occur reduced vitamin K is oxidised. Warfarin prevents the return of vitamin K to its reduced form.

1.58   Answers:

- A True
- B False
- C True
- D False
- E False

Warfarin is teratogenic in the first trimester. During the third trimester, it crosses the placenta and may result in fetal haemorrhage. Drugs that compete for plasma-binding sites (eg non-steroidal anti-inflammatory drugs) or inhibit its metabolism potentiate the effect of warfarin. The following drugs inhibit metabolism of warfarin: alcohol, allopurinol, erythromycin, ciprofloxacin, metronidazole and tricyclic antidepressants. The following drugs increase the metabolism of warfarin: barbiturates, rifampicin and carbamazepine.

1.59   Aprotinin:

☐ A Is derived from bovine lung

☐ B Inhibits plasmin

☐ C May be useful for the treatment of haemorrhage secondary to hyperplasminaemia

☐ D Increases the risk of deep vein thrombosis

☐ E Is a proteolytic enzyme inhibitor

1.60   Tranexamic acid:

☐ A Directly inhibits plasmin

☐ B Is more than 50% metabolised in the liver

☐ C Can be used in menorrhagia

☐ D Dosage needs altering with renal impairment

☐ E Is used in thromboembolic disease

1.59 Answers:

- A True
- B True
- C True
- D False
- E True

Aprotinin is a proteolytic enzyme inhibitor. It acts on trypsin, plasmin (at low doses) and tissue kallikrein (at high doses). It may also preserve platelet membrane-binding receptors. It is used as a blood conserver during open-heart surgery and liver transplantation. It may also be helpful in cases of haemorrhage due to hyperplasminaemia, eg during dissection of malignant tumours, in acute promyelocytic therapy and following thrombotic therapy.

Reference: *British National Formulary 52*. September 2006.

1.60 Answers:

- A False
- B False
- C True
- D True
- E False

Tranexamic acid inhibits plasminogen activation, not plasmin directly. It is 95% excreted unchanged in urine. It is used in menorrhagia (initially when menstruation has started), hereditary angioneurotic oedema and epistaxis. It is used in bleeding conditions in the presence of excess fibrinolysis. As it prevents fibrinolysis, it is prothrombotic and therefore contraindicated in thromboembolic disease.

1.61   Recombinant factor VIIa (rFVIIa):

☐ A Its main method of action is replacement of deficient factor VII

☐ B Causes a generalised systemic procoagulant effect

☐ C Has a half-life of 30 minutes in normal controls

☐ D Has pH as the key indicator of the likelihood of success of treatment

☐ E Can activate factor X

1.61   Answers:

- A False
- B False
- C False
- D True
- E True

rFVIIa is formed using recombinant DNA technology. It has a half-life of 2–3 hours in both normal controls and patients suffering with haemophilia. This may be shorter in the bleeding patient. Although it does provide additional factor VII, this is not its main method of action. It causes activation of coagulation with thrombin generation (by tissue factor-dependent and -independent pathways) and factor X activation.

It is thought not to cause a generalised systemic procoagulant effect; instead the action is localised to the site of vessel damage. Although pH is the main determinant of treatment success (with acidotic conditions inhibiting its action), currently there is no evidence that reversal of acidosis before treatment improves outcome. It is probably a marker of the extreme physiological state of the patient.

Reference: A critical appraisal of the use of recombinant factor VIIa in acquired bleeding conditions. *British Journal of Haematology* 2006; 133: 355–63.

1.62   Regarding the drugs used for postoperative nausea and vomiting:

☐ A Drugs acting on the chemosensitive trigger zone (CTZ) must first cross the blood–brain barrier

☐ B Metoclopramide exerts its prokinetic effect by acting as an agonist at the 5-HT$_4$ receptor

☐ C Muscarinic antagonists act on receptors located in the hindbrain medulla

☐ D Histamine (H$_1$)-receptor antagonists have an effect on the vestibular nucleus

☐ E Ondansetron antagonises gut and brain 5-HT$_3$ receptors

1.62   Answers:

- A False
- B True
- C True
- D True
- E True

The CTZ is situated outside the blood–brain barrier. Metoclopramide exerts a prokinetic effect on the stomach and upper gastrointestinal tract by acting as an agonist at 5-HT$_4$ receptors. At higher doses it also manifests 5-HT$_3$ antagonist function. H$_1$-receptors and muscarinic receptors are in the vomiting centre and the vestibular nucleus.

Reference: Physiology and pharmacology of nausea and vomiting. *Anaesthesia and Intensive Care Medicine* 2003; 4: 349–52.

1.63   Thiopental:

☐ A   Is 50% protein bound

☐ B   Is more potent than methohexital

☐ C   Forms an acidic solution when dissolved in water

☐ D   Is stored under nitrogen (not air) to prevent acidification by atmospheric carbon dioxide

☐ E   Is stored with sodium carbonate to reduce its acidification

1.64   Thiopental:

☐ A   Has an incidence of anaphylaxis of 1 per 1000 exposures

☐ B   Is relatively contraindicated in porphyria

☐ C   Has a volume of distribution greater than that of propofol

☐ D   Has a pK_a of 10.5

☐ E   In solution is bacteriostatic

1.63 Answers:

- A False
- B False
- C False
- D True
- E True

Thiopental is 80% protein bound and less potent than methohexital. In water it forms an alkaline solution with pH 10.5. The undissociated acid is insoluble so, to prevent its formation, sodium carbonate 6% is added to prevent hydrogen ion build-up and it is stored under nitrogen.

1.64 Answers:

- A False
- B False
- C False
- D False
- E True

Anaphylaxis is seen in 1 : 20 000 exposures. Porphyric crisis can be precipitated by thiopental and therefore it is an absolute contraindication, particularly as other intravenous induction agents are safe, including propofol.

It is presented as a sodium salt with a pK_a of 7.6. Once dissolved in water it forms an alkaline solution with pH 10.5. Remember that all salts of weak acids are alkaline in solution. It is stable and as it is bacteriostatic it can be stored for a few days.

It has a volume of distribution of 2.5 l/kg compared with 4.0 l/kg for propofol.

1.65 Thiopental:

- ☐ A In low doses is analgesic
- ☐ B Causes decrease in antidiuretic hormone (ADH)
- ☐ C Causes decrease in central nervous system (CNS) carbon dioxide production
- ☐ D Forms insoluble crystals when injected intra-arterially
- ☐ E Acidotic patients need less thiopental for the same effect

1.66 2,6-Diisopropylphenol:

- ☐ A Is a weak acid
- ☐ B Has a pK_a of 7.6
- ☐ C Has a greater clearance (ml/kg/min) when compared with thiopental
- ☐ D Has an elimination half-life similar to that of etomidate
- ☐ E Has protein binding similar to ketamine

1.65   Answers:

- A   False
- B   False
- C   True
- D   True
- E   True

At very low doses thiopental is actually antanalgesic. It causes an increase in ADH release secondary to its depressive effects on the cardiovascular system. A decrease in cardiac output also leads to a decrease in urine output. Thiopental reduces brain activity and therefore decreases oxygen consumption and CO_2 production. Insoluble crystals form in both venous and arterial systems; however, the collateral venous supply dilutes these crystals. Crystal formation in the arterial system can lead to distal infarction. Thiopental is a weak acid; with a decrease in pH there is an increase in free unionised drug and therefore it has a greater response.

1.66   Answers:

- A   True
- B   False
- C   True
- D   False
- E   False

Propofol (2,6-diisopropylphenol) is a weak acid with a pK_a of 11 and almost entirely unionised at physiological pH. It has a clearance of 30–60 ml/kg per min compared with 3.5 ml/kg per min for thiopental. It has an elimination half-life of 5–12 hours compared with etomidate 1–4 hours. Around 25% of ketamine is protein bound compared with almost 100% of propofol.

1.67 The following intravenous induction agents have active metabolites:

☐ A Thiopental

☐ B Propofol

☐ C Etomidate

☐ D Ketamine

☐ E Methohexital

1.68 Propofol:

☐ A Can be associated with CNS excitatory effects in 10% of patients

☐ B Reduces myocardial contractility

☐ C May turn urine green

☐ D Is predominantly protein bound to α_1-acid glycoprotein

☐ E Has glucuronide as its main metabolite

1.67   Answers:

- A   True
- B   False
- C   False
- D   True
- E   True

Methohexital has minimally active metabolites. Norketamine (the active metabolite of ketamine) is thought to be 30% as potent as ketamine.

1.68   Answers:

- A   True
- B   True
- C   True
- D   False
- E   False

As a weak acid, propofol is predominantly bound to albumin. The main metabolites are a quinol (approximately 60%) and a glucuronide (approximately 40%).

The decrease in cardiac output may be due to a decrease in contractility, a reduction in systemic vascular resistance or a combination of the two (dependent upon which book you read!).

1.69 Ketamine:

☐ A *R* enantiomer is the more potent when compared with the *S* enantiomer

☐ B Can be given intramuscularly for purposes of induction

☐ C Acts at many receptors including *N*-methyl-ᴅ-aspartic acid (NMDA) receptors

☐ D Is a sympathetic stimulant

☐ E Can be given rectally for sedation

1.70 Ketamine:

☐ A Is helpful in managing bronchoconstriction

☐ B When given intravenously becomes effective after one arm–brain circulation time

☐ C Alters the α-wave on an EEG

☐ D Acts on GABA receptors

☐ E Has a significant antiepileptic effect

1.69 Answers:

- A False
- B True
- C True
- D True
- E True

Ketamine is presented as a racemic mixture of two enantiomers. S^+ and R^- of which S is three to four times more potent. It forms an acidic solution in water with pH 3.5–5.5. It can be administered orally, rectally, intravenously, intramuscularly, intrathecally or epidurally (if preservative free). It increases circulating levels of norepinephrine and epinephrine and therefore increases cardiac output, heart rate, blood pressure and myocardial oxygen requirement.

1.70 Answers:

- A True
- B False
- C True
- D False
- E False

Ketamine is a sympathetic stimulant and therefore produces bronchodilatation along with other cardiovascular effects. The intravenously administered preparation takes approximately 90 seconds to have an effect. It causes an increase in cerebral oxygen consumption and blood flow. α-Waves are replaced by θ- and δ-waves. It does not affect the GABA receptor. It is thought to act on NMDA, 5-HT and opioid receptors. It has no antiepileptic effect but nor is it epileptogenic.

1.71   With regard to etomidate:

☐   A   Its initial effect is terminated by rapid redistribution into tissues

☐   B   Both etomidate and cimetidine are derived from similar structural groups

☐   C   It has an increased incidence of nausea and vomiting when compared with propofol

☐   D   It is safe to use in patients with porphyria

☐   E   It is more than 50% protein bound

1.72   Morphine:

☐   A   Strictly speaking is an opiate

☐   B   Is routinely used for intrathecal analgesia in the UK

☐   C   Has its peak effect within 5 minutes of intravenous bolus

☐   D   Reduces the cerebral sensitivity to hypoxia more than it reduces cerebral sensitivity to hypercapnia

☐   E   Causes pruritus that is most marked following intrathecal or epidural administration

1.71 Answers:

- A True
- B True
- C True
- D False
- E True

Etomidate is an imidazole derivative (like cimetidine). It is commonly used as an intravenous induction agent when cardiovascular stability is of importance. Its initial actions are terminated secondary to distribution into tissues. It is metabolised by hepatic esterases and plasma cholinesterase, and then renally excreted. Around 75% is protein bound to albumin. It, like thiopental, is contraindicated in porphyria. Propofol may have antiemetic properties, particularly when given without opioids.

1.72 Answers:

- A True
- B False
- C True
- D False
- E True

An opiate is a naturally occurring substance. Codeine, morphine and papaverine are all opiates as they are constituents of raw opium. Opioid is the broad term for substances both naturally occurring and synthetic, with affinity for the opioid receptor. Morphine is not routinely used for intrathecal analgesia (in the UK) as it can cause delayed respiratory depression secondary to its low lipid solubility. It affects the cerebral response to both hypoxia and hypercapnia but the latter is most markedly affected.

1.73 Morphine:

☐ A Given orally is absorbed in the stomach

☐ B Of all the opioids it is the least extensively protein bound

☐ C Is the least lipid soluble of all the commonly used opioids

☐ D Has a pK_a of 7.6

☐ E 6-Glucuronide is as potent as morphine

1.74 Diamorphine:

☐ A Is an opiate

☐ B Has a plasma half-life of approximately 5 minutes

☐ C Initially undergoes conjugation to become its active products

☐ D Is poorly absorbed orally

☐ E Is more protein bound than remifentanil

1.73   Answers:

- A False
- B True
- C True
- D False
- E False

Morphine (a weak base) is absorbed in its unionised form in the small intestine (in an alkaline environment). However, only 25% will reach the systemic circulation secondary to extensive first-pass metabolism. It has a pK_a of 8 compared with that of diamorphine at 7.6. Morphine has two major metabolites: morphine 3-glucuronide (accounting for ~70%) and morphine 6-glucuronide. The latter is over 10 times as potent as morphine.

1.74   Answers:

- A False
- B True
- C False
- D False
- E False

Diamorphine is not a naturally occurring opiate and is a prodrug. It has no effect on opioid receptors until it has undergone (rapid) ester hydrolysis to 6-monoacetylmorphine and then liver metabolism to morphine. Its oral absorption is good owing to its good lipid solubility. However, it undergoes extensive first-past metabolism. It is 40% protein bound compared with 70% for remifentanil.

1.75 Methadone:
- [ ] A Has high first-pass metabolism
- [ ] B May prolong the QT interval in susceptible patients
- [ ] C Is approximately 50% excreted unchanged in urine
- [ ] D Undergoes metabolism to predominantly inactive metabolites
- [ ] E Excretion is enhanced by acidification of urine

1.76 Pethidine:
- [ ] A Has an epileptogenic metabolite
- [ ] B May be administered in an unlimited fashion by midwifery staff
- [ ] C Is less lipid soluble than norpethidine
- [ ] D Is safe in renal failure
- [ ] E Is not safe to take in combination with lofepramine

1.75 Answers:

- A False
- B True
- C True
- D True
- E True

Methadone is a synthetic opioid which when taken orally is well absorbed, has a low first-pass metabolism and as such has a high oral bioavailability. It is less sedating and acts for longer periods than morphine. With prolonged use maximum twice-daily administration avoids accumulation. It can prolong the QT interval and monitoring is recommended for patients with hepatic or cardiac disease, electrolyte abnormalities, or concomitant treatment with QT-prolonging preparations. Monitoring is also recommended for patients taking >100 mg/day.

Reference: *British National Formulary 52*. September 2006.

1.76 Answers:

- A True
- B False
- C False
- D False
- E False

Pethidine is metabolised both by ester hydrolysis (yielding pethidinic acid) and by *N*-demethylation (yielding norpethidine). Norpethidine is less lipid soluble than pethidine. It accumulates in renal failure and is associated with hallucinations and grand mal seizures. Pethidine can be administered by midwives, a maximum of two doses, following which a doctor's prescription is needed (this policy may vary slightly in different units). Pethidine should not be administered with monoamine oxidase inhibitors; however, it can be administered with tricyclic antidepressants (eg lofepramine).

1.77   Pethidine:

☐ A   Accumulates in the fetus secondary to ion trapping

☐ B   Reaches peak fetal levels approximately 4 hours after maternal intramuscular administration

☐ C   Has a lower plasma protein binding when compared with alfentanil

☐ D   Has a higher unionised fraction at physiological pH when compared with morphine

☐ E   Has a 30 times higher lipid solubility than morphine

1.78   Alfentanil:

☐ A   Has a pK_a of 7.2

☐ B   Has significantly lower lipid solubility than fentanyl

☐ C   Has a half-life that is increased with concomitant midazolam administration

☐ D   Undergoes acetylation to form its metabolites

☐ E   Metabolites are renally excreted

1.77   Answers:

- A   True
- B   True
- C   True
- D   False
- C   True

As pethidine is a base, in a more acidic environment it becomes ionised and therefore becomes trapped in the fetus. Pethidine is approximately 60% plasma protein bound when compared with the 90% plasma protein binding of alfentanil. At physiological pH pethidine is only ~5% unionised compared with ~20% of morphine.

1.78   Answers:

- A   False
- B   True
- C   True
- D   False
- E   True

Alfentanil has a pK_a of 6.5. Fentanyl is approximately six times more lipid soluble than alfentanil. It is metabolised in the liver (*N*-demethylation) by CYP3A3/4 enzymes, as is midazolam, and therefore its elimination can be reduced with concomitant administration. Metabolites are conjugated and excreted renally.

1.79   Alfentanil:

☐ A Has an elimination half-life greater than fentanyl

☐ B Has lipid solubility greater than remifentanil

☐ C Has a volume of distribution less than fentanyl

☐ D Has a unionised fraction at physiological pH that exceeds that of remifentanil

☐ E Has a clearance less than morphine

1.79   Answers:

- A   False
- B   True
- C   True
- D   True
- E   True

Alfentanil has an elimination half-life of 100 min, a clearance of 6 ml/kg per min, a volume of distribution of 0.6 l/kg and a pK_a of 6.5. (Remember all the 6s.) At physiological pH it is 89% unionised compared with remifentanil, which is 68% unionised.

Alfentanil has a rapid speed of action; this is owing to its relatively low pK_a, which renders it ~90% unionised at physiological pH.

Fentanyl has an elimination half-life of 190 min, a clearance of 13 ml/kg per min, a volume of distribution of 4 l/kg and a pK_a of 8.4.

1.80   Regarding opioids:

☐   A   Fentanyl is the most rapidly cleared of all the opioids used in common practice

☐   B   Fentanyl carries no risk of respiratory depression when used to augment neuroaxial blockade

☐   C   A 25-µg fentanyl patch is the equivalent of 40 mg morphine salt daily

☐   D   20 mg Oramorph is roughly equivalent to 20 mg oxycodone (orally)

☐   E   3 mg diamorphine intramuscularly is roughly equivalent to 10 mg morphine orally

1.80   Answers:

- A   False
- B   False
- C   False
- D   False
- E   True

Fentanyl can cause respiratory depression when used with neuroaxial blockade as can diamorphine, but to a lesser degree than morphine, which has low lipid solubility and therefore produces a higher incidence of delayed respiratory depression. Of all the opioids, remifentanil has the most rapid clearance at 40 ml/kg per min.

Equivalent conversions for fentanyl patch from morphine are as follows:

Morphine salt – mg daily	Fentanyl patch μcg – (micrograms) equivalent
90	25
180	50
270	75
360	100

Equivalent single doses (which is an approximate guide offered by the *British National Formulary* (BNF)):

- morphine salt (po)   10 mg
- diamorphine (im)   3 mg
- oxycodone (po)   5 mg

Reference: *British National Formulary 52*. September 2006

1.81   Regarding isomers:

☐   A   They are molecules with the same atomic formulas

☐   B   Structural isomers have identical bonds between atoms

☐   C   Morphine demonstrates tautomerism

☐   D   Prednisolone and aldosterone are structural isomers

☐   E   At physiological pH midazolam exists in an open configuration

1.81   Answers:

- A   True
- B   False
- C   True
- D   True
- E   False

Although isomers have the same atomic formulas, they have different structural forms. Structural isomers have different bonds between molecules. These different bonds can confer very dissimilar pharmacological properties, eg dihydrocodeine and dobutamine!

Tautomerism is a phenomenon whereby a molecule takes on different structural forms depending on, for example, their physical environment. This is well illustrated by midazolam. In acid conditions, it is ionised but when at physiological pH its ring structure closes and it becomes a lipophilic, unionised molecule.

1.82   The following are true of the pharmacology of old age:

☐ A Lipophilic drugs have a shorter elimination half-life in elderly people

☐ B Metaraminol may be a more effective hypertensive agent when compared with ephedrine

☐ C Elderly people need increased doses of non-depolarising muscle relaxants for effective paralysis

☐ D Elderly people have an increased number of extra-junctional cholinergic receptors

☐ E Inhalational induction is less rapid in elderly people

Pharmacology MCQs

1.82   Answers:

- A   False
- B   True
- C   False
- D   True
- E   True

With age, comes an increase in body lipid content. This increases the volume of distribution of lipophilic drugs and, when compounded by the reduction in organ-based elimination, it increases their elimination half-life and duration of action.

β-receptors are not as sensitive in elderly people and, as such, atropine and ephedrine may not be as effective. α-receptors on arteries and veins are still sensitive and so metaraminol is still as effective. Elderly people have more extra-junctional receptors but they have a decreased metabolism of drugs and therefore the usual dose of non-depolarising muscle relaxant can be given provided that more time is allowed for the drug to work. Due to increased ventilation–perfusion mismatching and closing capacity, achievement of tidal volume inhalational induction takes longer.

Reference: Perioperative care of the elderly. *Continuing Education in Anaesthesia, Critical Care and Pain* 2004; 4: 193–6.

1.83   Regarding local anaesthetics for spinal anaesthesia:

☐ A   A hyperbaric solution has a baricity > 1.0010

☐ B   A hypobaric solution has a baricity < 0.9990

☐ C   Addition of alcohol to a solution will render it hyperbaric

☐ D   Dropping the temperature of plain bupivacaine to 5°C makes it behave like a hyperbaric solution in the cerebrospinal fluid (CSF)

☐ E   Glucose solutions as low as 2% are considered hyperbaric

1.84   Regarding intrathecal anaesthesia:

☐ A   Solutions containing vasoconstrictors have significantly reduced mean spread compared with those without

☐ B   Alkalisation of solutions increases speed of onset

☐ C   Posture influences speed of isobaric solutions in the CSF

☐ D   A 20° head-down tilt will cause a significant increase in the mean spread of a hyperbaric solution

☐ E   It is thought that intrathecal local anaesthetic appears to stop spreading approximately 20–25 minutes after injection

1.83   Answers:

- A True
- B True
- C False
- D True
- E True

Alcohol and strychnine were used in intrathecal anaesthesia to render solutions hypobaric; however, neurotoxicity affected their continued use. Normal glucose solutions of 5% are used in intrathecal anaesthesia for its hyperbaric effect. Evidence shows that glucose levels as low as 0.8% produce a solution that behaves in a hyperbaric fashion.

Reference: Intrathecal drug spread. *British Journal of Anaesthesia* 2004; 93(4): 568–78.

1.84   Answers:

- A False
- B False
- C False
- D False
- E True

Solutions with and without vasoconstrictors have the same spread although the duration of action is altered. Alkalinisation of the local anaesthetic again has no effect on speed but may affect duration of block. Isobaric solution spread is not influenced by position. Studies show that even a 30° cephalad tilt only minimally affects the mean spread of a hyperbaric solution; however, it does increase variability. Although spread appears to stop 20–25 minutes post injection, marked changes in a patient's position up to 2 hours after injection can lead to significant changes in extent of the block. This is thought to be independent of the baricity and is likely to be secondary to bulk movement of CSF that still contains a high concentration of local anaesthetic.

Reference: Intrathecal drug spread. *British Journal of Anaesthesia* 2004; 93(4): 568–78.

1.85   Pulmonary vascular resistance (PVR) is increased by:

☐ A   Norepinephrine

☐ B   Histamine

☐ C   5-HT

☐ D   Acetylcholine

☐ E   Prostacyclin

1.86   The following are true of drug metabolism by the lungs:

☐ A   Prostacyclin (PGI_2) is not metabolised by the lungs

☐ B   Prostaglandins (eg PGE_2) are removed by the lung

☐ C   Leukotrienes are unaffected by the lung

☐ D   Norepinephrine is partially removed by the lung

☐ E   Bradykinin is largely inactivated by the lung

1.85   Answers:

- A   True
- B   True
- C   True
- D   False
- E   False

A helpful pneumonic to remember agents that decrease PVR is **PIANO**: **P**rostacyclin, **I**soprenaline, **A**cetylcholine, **N**itric oxide and **O**xygen.

1.86   Answers:

- A   True
- B   True
- C   False
- D   True
- E   True

PGE_2, $PGF_{2\alpha}$, leukotrienes and 5-HT are almost completely removed by the lung. PGI_2 and PGA_2 and PGA_1 are unaffected by the lung. Up to 30% of norepinephrine is removed by the lung. Epinephrine, angiotensin II and ADH are not significantly affected by passage through the lung.

Reference: West, JB. *Respiratory Physiology – the Essentials*. 7th edn. Philadelphia: Lippincott Williams and Wilkins, 2004

1.87 **Regarding drugs affecting calcium homoeostasis:**

☐ A Glucocorticoids inhibit osteoclast activity

☐ B They may have an anti-vitamin D action

☐ C Growth hormone increases calcium urinary excretion

☐ D Thyroid hormone can cause hypocalcaemia

☐ E Insulin increases bone formation

1.88 **Amiodarone:**

☐ A Has solely class IV actions (Vaughan–Williams classification)

☐ B Is extensively protein bound

☐ C Has metabolites with some anti-arrhythmic action

☐ D Has a low oral bioavailability

☐ E Decreases the refractory period of myocardial action potentials

1.87 Answers:

- A True
- B True
- C True
- D True
- E True

Glucocorticoids inhibit osteoclast formation and activity; over long periods they also cause osteoporosis by decreasing bone formation and increasing bone resorption. Growth hormone does increase calcium urinary excretion but it also causes increased calcium intestinal absorption with a resultant positive calcium balance. People with untreated diabetes have significant bone loss as insulin increases bone formation.

Reference: Calcium homeostasis. *RCOA Bulletin* 2003; 18: 883–6.

1.88 Answers:

- A False
- B True
- C True
- D False
- E False

Amiodarone is a useful anti-arrhythmic for SVT (supraventricular tachycardia) and VT. Although classified as having class III activity it also demonstrates class I, II and IV activity. Its blocking effect on the potassium channel causes a prolongation of phase 3 (repolarisation). This lengthens the action potential and the refractory period. The oral bioavailability is 50–70%. It is 95% plasma protein bound and is hepatically metabolised to desmethylamiodarone, which has some anti-arrhythmic activity.

1.89   Regarding lidocaine toxicity:

☐ A Toxicity occurs with blood concentrations over 4 μg/ml

☐ B CNS toxicity is an early sign of intravenous overdose

☐ C Cardiac arrest precedes respiratory arrest

☐ D The maximum recommended infiltration dose of plain 2% lidocaine in a 70 kg man is 30 ml

☐ E It is more likely in the presence of liver failure

1.90   Regarding the metabolism of sodium nitroprusside:

☐ A Reaction in the red blood cell causes release of CN^- and methaemoglobin

☐ B CN^- combines with vitamin B_{12} to yield toxic thiocyanate

☐ C Rhodanase enzyme is found only in the liver

☐ D Red blood cells can liberate CN^- from thiocyanate via the enzyme thiocyanate oxidase

☐ E Thiocyanate and CN^- are equally toxic to cytochrome oxidase

1.89 **Answers:**

- A True
- B True
- C False
- D False
- E True

Lidocaine toxicity can be viewed as plasma concentrations:

- >4 µg/ml – circumoral tingling, tinnitus, dizziness, paraesthesia
- 10 µg/ml – loss of consciousness, convulsions
- 15 µg/ml – coma, stroke, myocardial depression
- 20 µg/ml – cardiac arrhythmia, respiratory arrest
- 25 µg/ml – ventricular arrest.

Toxic doses are 3 mg/kg of plain solution or 7 mg/kg of lidocaine with epinephrine. A 2% solution contains 20 mg/ml. Therefore, a 70 kg man should receive an upper limit of 10.5 ml 2% lidocaine. This is the recommended dose. Lidocaine undergoes hepatic metabolism and therefore will present increased risk of toxicity in patients with hepatic failure.

Reference: Urquhart, Blunt and Pinnock. *The Anaesthesia Viva 1 (Physiology and Pharmacology).* 2nd edn.

1.90 **Answers:**

- A True
- B False
- C False
- D True
- E False

Sodium nitroprusside enters red blood cells and combines with oxyhaemoglobin to form five CN^- ions and methaemoglobin. CN^- and methaemoglobin form cyanomethaemoglobin (non-toxic). CN^- ions react with sulphydryl groups in liver and renal tissue secondary to the enzyme action of rhodanase. Thiocyanate is produced, which is 100 times less toxic than CN^-. Thiocyanate is excreted renally with an elimination half-life of 2 days. It can also be converted to CN^- by thiocyanate oxidase found in red blood cells.

1.91   Regarding the treatment of sodium nitroprusside toxicity:

☐ A   Plasma CN^- > 8 µg/ml results in toxicity

☐ B   Dicobalt edetate chelates CN^- ions so decreasing toxicity

☐ C   Sodium nitrate increases available methaemoglobin so producing more thiocyanate

☐ D   Vitamin B_{12} is most effective as a prophylactic agent

☐ E   Sodium thiosulphate decreases CN^- ions by increasing thiocyanate production

1.92   Phosphodiesterase inhibitor aminophylline:

☐ A   Inhibits all five phosphodiesterase isoenzymes

☐ B   Blocks the adenosine receptor on mast cells, inhibiting degranulation

☐ C   Reduces seizure threshold

☐ D   Causes fluid retention

☐ E   Elimination is reduced by phenytoin

1.91   Answers:

- A True
- B True
- C False
- D True
- E True

Sodium nitrate and amyl nitrate cause an increase in methaemoglobin, so providing more substrate for the production of non-toxic cyanomethaemoglobin. Vitamin B_{12} combines with CN^- to form cyanocobalamin which is also non-toxic but of little value in the acute setting.

1.92   Answers:

- A True
- B True
- C True
- D False
- E False

Aminophylline is a non-selective phosphodiesterase inhibitor. It prevents tubular sodium reabsorption and is therefore a diuretic. It is metabolised via the cytochrome P450 system. As phenytoin induces this system it therefore increases elimination.

1.93 Diazoxide:

☐ A Is a diuretic

☐ B Causes hyperuricaemia

☐ C Causes hypoglycaemia

☐ D Is used to treat hypertensive crises associated with renal disease

☐ E Effect on blood sugar lasts longer than its effect on blood pressure

1.94 Regarding anticholinergics:

☐ A Hyoscine crosses the blood–brain barrier

☐ B Only the L-atropine isomer is active

☐ C Glycopyrrolate is a quaternary amine

☐ D Glycopyrrolate is predominantly excreted unchanged in the urine

☐ E Atropine may cause transient bradycardia

1.93   Answers:

- A False
- B True
- C False
- D True
- E True

Related to the thiazide diuretics chemically, it may be confusing to find that it actually causes a reduction in urine output secondary to an increase in renin and aldosterone. Diazoxide causes decreased insulin secretion, which can be used to treat hypoglycaemia. It also causes arterial vasodilatation (secondary to increased cAMP effect in arterioles), which is useful for the treatment of hypertensive crises. While producing arterial vasodilatation, it also increases catecholamine release, causing an increase in heart rate and cardiac output. Its hypoglycaemic effects last approximately 8 hours compared with its effects on blood pressure, which last 5 hours. Oral bioavailability is 80% and it is 90% protein bound.

1.94   Answers:

- A True
- B True
- C True
- D True
- E True

Hyoscine and atropine are tertiary amines and are therefore able to cross the blood–brain barrier, unlike glycopyrrolate (a quaternary amine). 80% of glycopyrrolate is excreted unchanged in the urine. Atropine may cause a transient bradycardia reflecting its partial agonist effect at cardiac muscarinic receptors. Although present in a racemic mixture only the L-atropine isomer is active (as is the case with hyoscine).

1.95 Regarding chirality:

☐ A Stereoisomers have the same atomic structure but different bonds between molecules

☐ B Enantiomers are chemicals that are mirror images of each other

☐ C Levobupivacaine is an S^- enantiomer

☐ D The *R/S* (*rectus* or *sinister*) naming system reflects the direction of rotation of a plane of polarised light

☐ E Mivacurium is a geometrical isomer existing predominantly in the *cis–cis* configuration

1.96 Sympathomimetics – epinephrine:

☐ A Is used in doses of 1 ml/kg of 1 : 10 000 iv during paediatric asystolic arrests

☐ B At low doses can cause a fall in peripheral vascular resistance

☐ C When used with halothane, doses should be kept to within 100 µg/10 min to avoid arrhythmias

☐ D Metabolites are excreted in the urine as vanillylmandelic acid

☐ E At high doses, inhibits insulin secretion

1.95 Answers:

- A False
- B True
- C True
- D False
- E False

Option A refers to structural isomers. Stereoisomers have both the same atomic formulas and bonds but different arrangements around a chiral centre (or centres).

Option D describes the *dextro/levo* naming system with clockwise rotation of the polarised light being *dextro* (to the right) and anticlockwise rotation being *levo* (to the left). The *R/S* naming system refers to the orientation of molecules around a chiral centre, *R* standing for *rectus* and *S* for *sinister* (the Latin for right and left respectively). There is no link between the two naming systems. Levobupivacaine is an enantio-pure preparation, ie containing only one isomer. Most isometric drugs have helpful therapeutic properties conferred by the *sinister* enantiomer.

Mivacurium exists predominantly in the *trans–trans* form (~60%).

1.96 Answers:

- A False
- B True
- C True
- D True
- E True

Paediatric resuscitation doses for epinephrine are 0.1 ml/kg 1 : 10 000. At low doses, β effects predominate which decrease peripheral vascular resistance and increase insulin secretion. At high doses α effects predominate, causing vasoconstriction and a decrease in insulin secretion.

1.97   Pharmacokinetics – acute intermittent porphyria:

☐ A Can be precipitated by sulphonamide antibiotics

☐ B Is more common in eastern Europeans

☐ C Results from a deficiency in porphobilinogen

☐ D Attacks are more common in women than men

☐ E Attacks can present with gastrointestinal symptoms

1.98   Adverse drug reactions – examples of type A (or augmented) reactions to drugs include the following:

☐ A Tinnitus with aspirin

☐ B Hypoglycaemia with insulin

☐ C Malignant hyperthermia with suxamethonium

☐ D Ataxia with phenytoin

☐ E Acute intermittent porphyria with barbiturates

1.97 Answers:

- A True
- B False
- C False
- D True
- E True

Acute intermittent porphyria is an example of a familial variation in drug response that affects anaesthesia. It can be precipitated by barbiturate anaesthetics, anticonvulsants, sulphonamide antibiotics, ranitidine, diclofenac, hyoscine, clonidine and lidocaine, to name a few!

Attacks are more common in women and northern Europeans (Sweden). Attacks present with gastrointestinal symptoms of pain, diarrhoea and vomiting, neurological symptoms including muscle weakness, convulsions and tremor. It results from a deficiency of the enzyme porphobilinogen deaminase, which leads to the accumulation of the haem precursors δ-aminolaevulinic acid and porphobilinogen, initially in the liver

1.98 Answers:

- A True
- B True
- C False
- D True
- E False

One way to classify adverse drug reactions is as either type A or augmented or type B or bizarre. Type A reactions are common and are often related to the pharmacological effect of the drug. They are commonly dose related. They can be a primary reaction due to an exaggerated response to the drug, eg hypoglycaemia with insulin or a secondary reaction, not directly related to the desired effect, eg tinnitus with aspirin. Type B reactions are bizarre, unpredicted and not dose related. Examples of type B reactions include suxamethonium apnoea, malignant hyperthermia and hepatic porphyria.

Reference: Adverse drug reactions. *Anaesthesia and Intensive Care Medicine* 2005; 6: 245–50.

1.99   Regarding adverse drug reactions – hypersensitivity reactions:

☐   A   Type 1 hypersensitivity reactions with penicillin are mainly caused by their degradation products

☐   B   Presentation with bronchospasm results from leukotriene release in the lungs

☐   C   They can occur secondary to IgE, IgG or IgM activation

☐   D   They are classed as type IV in the case of haemolytic anaemia after methyldopa

☐   E   They are described as class II when resulting from soluble antigens combining with circulating antibodies

1.99   Answers:

- A True
- B True
- C True
- D False
- E False

Type of Reaction	Cause	Example
Type I hypersensitivity	Antigen + protein causes IgE antibody formation attached to mast cells	Degradation products of penicillin, insect stings, peanut
Type II hypersensitivity	Drug combines with proteins in cells, inducing formation of IgG of IgM antibodies	Methyldopa – haemolytic anaemia Carbimazole – leukopenia
Type III hypersensitivity	Soluble antigen reacts with circulating IgG antibody	Serum sickness Rheumatic disease
Type IV hypersensitivity	Macrophage ingestion + T-lymphocyte activation	Tuberculin reaction Contact dermatitis

Reference: Adverse drug reactions. *Anaesthesia and Intensive Care Medicine* 2005; 6: 245–50.

1.100 Bioavailability:

☐ A Is defined as the fraction of an oral dose of a drug that reaches the systemic circulation when compared with a standard route of administration (usually intravenous)

☐ B Of warfarin is increased with concomitant use of barbiturates

☐ C Of aminophylline is increased in smokers

☐ D Of a buccally administered drug is decreased secondary to first-pass metabolism

☐ E When plotting plasma concentration vs time of an oral and intravenous preparation of a drug, the bioavailability is given by the area under the curve of oral divided by the intravenous preparation

1.100 Answers:

- A True
- B False
- C False
- D False
- E True

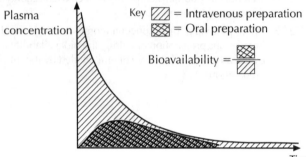

Figure: Bioavailability

Enzyme inducers increase the breakdown of the drug and therefore decrease the bioavailability, eg warfarin with barbiturates and aminophylline in smokers. Enzyme inhibition reduces drug breakdown therefore increasing the bioavailability of the drug, eg metronidazole with alcohol; intravenous, intramuscular, subcutaneous, transferral, sublingual, buccal and nasal drug administration avoid significant first-pass metabolism.

Enzyme inducers	Enzyme inhibitors
Barbiturates	Ecothiophate
Phenytoin	Metronidazole
Alcohol	Cimetidine
Smoking	Isoniazid
Rifampicin	Phenelzine

1.101   Drug distribution:

  A Of warfarin is almost entirely confined to the plasma

  B Of monoamines is negligible across the blood–brain barrier (BBB)

  C Is in general greater across a placenta when compared with a BBB

  D Between mother and fetus is affected by the drug's relative plasma acidity

  E Of highly protein bound drugs is very low

1.102   Drug metabolism:

  A By sulphation is an example of a phase I reaction

  B By acetylation occurs solely in the liver

  C In liver failure usually affects phase II metabolism before phase I

  D Of sevoflurane is by cytochrome P450 (isoform 2E1)

  E Of halothane is predominantly by reduction if the liver becomes hypoxic

1.101 Answers:

- A True
- B True
- C True
- D True
- E False

Warfarin is a highly protein-bound drug that is confined to the plasma as its unbound fraction is negligible. That is not to say that all highly protein bound drugs have minimal distribution. Propofol is 98% protein bound but has extensive distributions owing to the dynamic nature of the protein binding. The passage of monoamine across the BBB is negligible as it contains monoamine oxidases. The passage of drugs across a placenta is greater than across a BBB as it is less selective. Even moderately, lipid-soluble drugs can pass with ease. The drug distribution between mother and fetus can vary according to their plasma pH, eg pethidine will become more ionised in the lower pH of the fetal plasma, so leading to ion trapping.

1.102 Answers:

- A False
- B False
- C False
- D True
- E True

Phase I reactions include oxidation, reduction and hydrolysis. They are carried out by the mixed function oxidase system or the cytochrome P450 system within the endoplasmic reticulum. Other enzymes can also perform phase I metabolism, eg monoamine oxidases. Phase II reactions include glucuronidation, sulphation, acetylation, methylation and glycination. Phase II metabolism increases the water solubility of the drug so allowing excretion in bile and urine. Acetylation occurs in the liver, lung and spleen. Liver failure generally affects phase I reactions first.

1.103 Receptor agonists and antagonists. The following stems are correct in relation to the log dose–response curve illustrated:

☐ A Curve c could represent a partial agonist

☐ B Curve b could represent a drug that is less potent than that giving rise to curve a

☐ C Addition of a competitive antagonist to the drug giving curve a could lead to the dose–response curve c

☐ D The position of the curve on the abscissa denotes efficacy

☐ E Curve b could represent the action of phenoxybenzamine at the α-receptor

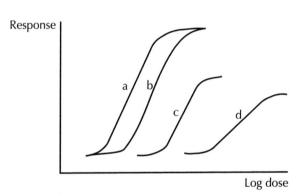

Figure: Log dose–response curves

1.103   Answers:

- A True
- B True
- C False
- D False
- E False

This sort of question is also easily examined in the viva. When interpreting these curves, remember, their position on the abscissa reflects potency, their maximal height reflects the efficacy and their slope is influenced by the number of receptors that must be activated to achieve that response. Note that the dictionary definition of abscissa: the shortest distance from a point to the vertical or *y* axis, measured parallel to the horizontal or *x* axis, ie the closer to the *y* axis, the more potent. The dose–response curves a and b represent full agonists, the drug giving curve b being less potent than that giving curve a. The dose–response curve b could also represent the addition of a competitive agonist to the drug, giving rise to curve a. The addition of a non-competitive agonist to the drugs represented by curves a or b could lead to a dose–response curve d. Non-competitive agonists affect all aspects of the curve. Phenoxybenzamine is an insurmountable antagonist at the α-receptor, no amount of agonist will produce the full receptor effect.

Reference: Receptors, agonists and antagonists. *Anaesthesia and Intensive Care Medicine* 2004; 5: 350–2.

1.104 The following are true of receptors:

☐ A All subunits of a ligand-gated ion channel traverse the membrane

☐ B G-protein coupled make up the largest proportion of membrane-bound receptors

☐ C Cholera toxin causes persistent activation of the G-protein that stimulates adenylyl cyclase (Gs)

☐ D Thyroxine exerts its effect via membrane tyrosine kinase

☐ E Activity of a receptor is analogous to affinity

1.104 Answers:

- A True
- B True
- C True
- D False
- E False

Receptors can be divided broadly into:

- Ligand-gated ion channels eg nicotinic, GABA receptor
- G-protein linked, eg sympathomimetic receptors
- Direct enzyme linked, eg insulin, atrial naturetic peptide (ANP)
- Intracellular receptors affecting gene transcription, eg steroids, thyroxine

Ligand gated channels are multi-subunit receptors. All these subunits traverse the membrane. G-protein-coupled receptors are the largest group of membrane-bound receptors, (covered in Question 1.107). Thyroxine binds to an intracellular, nuclear, thyroid hormone receptor. Insulin binds to an extracellular receptor. Binding triggers the phosphorylation of tyrosine, by the intracellular portion of the receptor. This greatly increases the activity of tyrosine kinase, which in turn initiates insulin's intracellular effect. Affinity refers to how well a drug binds to a receptor. Activity refers to the extent of receptor activity caused by the drug binding.

Reference: Receptors, agonists and antagonists. *Anaesthesia and Intensive Care Medicine* 2004; 5: 350–2.

1.105   Drug binding:

☐   A   The stable heparin–antithrombin III complex is an example of a covalent bond

☐   B   Dipole–dipole interactions depend on van der Waals' forces

☐   C   Covalent bonds form following the transfer of electrons

☐   D   The hydroxyl group of edrophonium is attracted to the anionic site of acetylcholinesterase

☐   E   Albumin binds only neutral or acidic drugs

1.105   Answers:

- A   False
- B   True
- C   True
- D   False
- E   False

Ionic bonds are readily reversible bonds between ionised compounds and anionic and cationic sites on proteins. Heparin contains an anionic pentasaccharide group that is attracted to basic arginine residues in antithrombin III

Dipole–dipole interactions occur between molecules that are partially positive and others that are partially negatively charged. The strength of the bond depends on the distance between the molecules. The critical distance that yields the greatest attraction is called van der Waals' radius.

Hydrogen bonds are another example of dipole–dipole interactions. These occur between partially positive hydrogen atoms in hydroxyl or secondary amine groups and electronegative atoms with unshared electrons, eg oxygen. Edrophonium forms a hydrogen bond by its hydroxyl group at the esteratic site on acetylcholinesterase. Covalent bonds involve the sharing of electrons rather than complete transfer. Stable bonds are formed. Albumin predominantly binds acid and neutral drugs but also binds some basic drugs.

Reference: Bonding, binding and isomerism. *Anaesthesia and Intensive Care Medicine* 2004; 5: 345–8.

1.106   The following drugs are over 50% protein bound in plasma:

☐   A   Ropivacaine

☐   B   Warfarin

☐   C   Morphine

☐   D   Atenolol

☐   E   Phenytoin

1.106 Answers:

- A True
- B True
- C False
- D False
- E True

Drug	Percentage protein bound
Ropivacaine	94
Bupivacaine	95
Lidocaine	65
Atracurium	<20
Fentanyl	80
Alfentanil	90
Morphine	30
Pethidine	65
Warfarin	99
Phenytoin	95
Atenolol	5

Reference: Bonding, binding and isomerism. *Anaesthesia and Intensive Care Medicine* 2004; 5: 345–7.

1.107 The following are true regarding sympathomimetic G-coupled proteins:

☐ A α_1-Receptors are Gi coupled

☐ B β_2-Receptors are Gs coupled

☐ C All dopamine receptors are Gs coupled

☐ D Activation of Gs-coupled receptors increases cAMP action

☐ E Stimulation of Gq-coupled receptors decreases the activity of protein kinase C

1.107 Answers:

- A False
- B True
- C False
- D True
- E False

Receptor	G-coupled protein
α_1	Gq
α_2	Gi
β_1	Gs
β_2	Gs
β_3	Gs
D_1	Gs
D_2	Gi

Gs-coupled receptors cause stimulation of cAMP production. This in turn stimulates protein kinase A by binding to one of its sites (R or regulatory site). This causes its active site (C unit) to be revealed, which is responsible for its effects, including positive inotropic and chronotropic effect in the heart and relaxation of smooth muscle in the bronchi and vasculature by β_1- and β_2-receptors.

Gi-coupled proteins inhibit cAMP production. α_2-Receptors are an example. They are widespread in the CNS and a decreased cAMP causes sedation and analgesia.

Gq-coupled protein activation causes increased action of phospholipase C, causing the breakdown of phosphatidylinositol 4,5-bisphosphate (PIP_2) to inositol trisphosphate (IP_3) and diacylglycerol (DAG). IP_3 causes calcium release in the endoplasmic reticulum and DAG causes activation of protein kinase C. This increase in calcium causes its effects including vasoconstriction in vascular smooth muscle by α_1-receptor activation.

1.108 The following is true regarding pharmacokinetics in the obese patient:

☐ A Ideal body weight (IBW) is calculated by (height in cm – 100) for adult males

☐ B Lean body mass (LBM) is calculated using height, weight and sex

☐ C Below IBW, LBM and total body weight (TBW) are similar

☐ D Remifentanil shows a significant increase in volume of distribution in the obese patient

☐ E If a drug is hydrophilic, its dose should be calculated according to an obese patient's LBM

1.108 Answers:

- A True
- B True
- C True
- D False
- E True

IBW is calculated as shown:

IBW (kg) = height (cm) − x

(where $x = 100$ for adult men and 105 for adult women).

LBM can be calculated as shown:

Male LBM = 1.1(weight) − 128(weight ÷ height)^2

or for female LBM = 1.07(weight) − 148(weight ÷ height)^2.

Highly lipophilic drugs show an increase in volume of distribution in the obese patient. Remifentanil is highly lipophilic; however, it shows no significant change in distribution in obese patients. As a result, the dosage should be calculated based on the IBW. The obese patient has an increase in LBM when compared with non-obese individuals by up to 20–40%. Therefore, when calculating the dosage of a hydrophilic drug, it is more accurate to correct the dose to the LBM than the IBW.

Reference: Pharmacokinetics in obese patients. *Continuing Education Anaesthesia, Critical Care and Pain* 2004; 4(5): 152–5.

1.109 The following are true concerning drugs in the obese patient:

☐ A Lipophilic propofol accumulates significantly

☐ B Maintenance dose of propofol can be calculated according to the TBW

☐ C The volume of distribution of midazolam increases in parallel with body weight

☐ D Suxamethonium dosage should be calculated from the IBW

☐ E Paracetamol dosage should be calculated based on the TBW

1.109 Answers:

- A False
- B True
- C True
- D False
- E False

Although lipophilic, propofol does not accumulate in obese patients. The maintenance dose can be calculated according to the actual body weight with no risk of accumulation, but this may cause significant haemodynamic sequelae. Various pharmacokinetic models have been developed to avoid this including:

Corrected weight = ideal body weight + (0.4 × excess weight)

(Gepts et al).

The volume of distribution and half-life of midazolam increase in parallel with body weight but the total metabolic clearance remains unchanged. Therefore, the rate of a continuous infusion of midazolam must be adjusted to the IBW. The dosage of suxamethonium should be calculated based on the TBW, as should mivacurium. Administration of normal doses of paracetamol to an obese patient yields the same plasma levels as in normal patients. Therefore, the dosage to IBW is safer.

Reference: Pharmacokinetics in obese patients. *Continuing Education in Anaesthesia, Critical Care and Pain*, British Journal of Anaesthesia 2004; 4(5): 152–5.

1.110 Regarding pharmacokinetics:

☐ A   The elimination rate constant (K) is the fraction by which the concentration of a drug reduces during a specified period

☐ B   The time constant is the time (measured from a point zero) at which the elimination of the drug would have been complete if the initial rate of elimination had continued

☐ C   A drug with a volume of distribution at steady state of 0.16 l/kg is likely to be highly ionised

☐ D   A unit of measurement for time constant is minutes

☐ E   The volume of distribution of fentanyl is significantly larger than propofol

1.110 Answers:

- A True
- B True
- C True
- D True
- E False

The elimination rate constant (K) is measured in units of time t^{-1}. The time constant corresponds to the time taken for the concentration to fall to 37% of its initial value. It is measured in the unit time. Highly ionised drugs do not readily cross lipid membranes and so have a low volume of distribution, eg glycopyrrolate with a V_d 0.16 l/kg. Fentanyl and propofol have similar volumes of distribution at 4 l/kg.

1.111 Pharmacokinetics:

- ☐ A Absorption of weakly acidic drugs is facilitated by high pH
- ☐ B Dopamine is metabolised in the gut mucosa
- ☐ C After an intravenous drug administration, high cardiac output causes a higher peak blood concentration (when compared with a lower cardiac output state)
- ☐ D The rapid redistribution of thiopental is known as the α phase
- ☐ E At high concentrations aspirin can undergo zero-order kinetics.

1.111 Answers:

- A False
- B True
- C False
- D True
- E True

Acids become more unionised in an acidic environment. Bases become more ionised in acidic conditions:

$A^- + H^+ \rightarrow AH$

$B + H^+ \rightarrow BH^+$.

If an intravenous drug is given to a patient with a high cardiac output state, the drug is diluted by the volume of blood; this leads to a lower plasma concentration. The rapid emergence from anaesthesia after an initial intravenous bolus of thiopental is a result of the α phase. Initially the thiopental is concentrated in the fat-soluble tissue with a rich blood supply including the brain. However, as the less well-perfused tissues absorb more of the drug, the plasma concentration drops and therefore the drug leaves the brain and enters the plasma down the concentration gradient. The fall in brain concentration leads to emergence from anaesthesia.

First-order kinetics occurs in non-saturated enzyme reactions. Elimination is dependent on the concentration of the drug and is exponential. Zero-order kinetics occur in saturated enzyme systems. The amount of drug eliminated is constant per unit time and is limited by the enzyme action. At low concentrations, a drug can undergo first-order kinetics, but as the enzyme system becomes saturated, the elimination kinetics can change to zero order, eg aspirin.

1.112 Aspirin:

☐ A Absorption is greater in the stomach than in the small intestine

☐ B Is preferentially excreted in acidic urine

☐ C Has a pK_a of 6

☐ D Is predominantly unionised at physiological pH

☐ E Is predominantly bound to albumin in the systemic circulation

1.112 Answers:

- A False
- B False
- C False
- D False
- E True

Aspirin is an acid with a pK_a of 3. In the acid environment of the stomach, it is in its unionised form, which may lead you to believe that its absorption would be greater than in the basic environment of the small intestine. The unionised aspirin, however, becomes ionised and trapped in the gastric mucosal cells preventing absorption into the systemic circulation. The large surface area of the small bowel means that the greater part of its absorption occurs here. Alkaline urine promotes its excretion, as more ionised molecules are excreted in urine. It is predominantly ionised at physiological pH. Remember:

$A^- + H^+ \rightarrow AH$.

It is 85% protein bound in the plasma, mainly to albumin.

1.113 The volume of distribution (V_d):

☐ A Is the plasma concentration divided by the initial dose

☐ B Of a drug that is confined to the extracellular space is approximately 14 litres

☐ C Of diazepam exceeds total body water

☐ D Divided by the clearance gives the rate constant for the exponential process of elimination

☐ E Is equal to the time constant divided by the clearance

1.113 Answers:

- A False
- B True
- C True
- D False
- E False

The volume of distribution (V_d) of a drug is the dose of drug divided by the plasma concentration. A drug with a low V_d that is highly protein bound and low lipid solubility will be largely confined to plasma. A lipid-soluble drug that is concentrated in tissues, eg diazepam, will have a large V_d (1–1.5 l/kg). Some equations to aid calculation of V_d are shown

$K = $ clearance $\div V_d$

Time constant $= 1 \div K = V_d \div$ clearance

where K is the rate constant for the exponential process of elimination of a drug.

1.114 Clearance:

☐ A Of a drug is given in the units ml/min

☐ B Of a drug by the liver is given by the product of hepatic blood flow and hepatic extraction ratio

☐ C Of a drug by the liver will depend predominantly on enzyme activity if the hepatic extraction ratio is >0.7

☐ D Of a drug by the kidneys that exceeds the glomerular filtration rate (GFR) is by both secretion and filtration

☐ E Of an unionised drug by the kidney is reduced secondary to tubular reabsorption

1.114 Answers:

- A True
- B True
- C False
- D True
- E True

Hepatic clearance = hepatic blood flow (ml/min) × hepatic extraction ratio.

If the drug has a high hepatic extraction ratio >0.7 then an alteration in hepatic blood flow will be the main determinant of clearance. This is termed perfusion-dependent elimination. If the hepatic extraction ratio is small (<0.3), then an increase in blood flow will have minimal effect, the main determinant of hepatic clearance being enzyme activity. This is termed 'capacity-dependent elimination'. Renal clearance is by both filtration and secretion. If a drug is unionised then it is able to pass freely into the renal tubules and therefore its renal clearance is reduced. This explains why altering the pH of urine, and therefore the percentage of unionised drug free to be absorbed, alter the clearance of a drug, eg aspirin and alkaline urine.

Reference: Modes of drug elimination and pharmacokinetic analysis. *Anaesthesia and Intensive Care Medicine* 2005; 6: 277–82.

1.115   Pharmacokinetics of inhaled anaesthetics. The following will increase the alveolar partial pressure (P_A):

☐   A   High alveolar ventilation

☐   B   A large functional reserve capacity (FRC)

☐   C   A high cardiac output

☐   D   A low blood : gas partition coefficient

☐   E   A high oil : gas partition coefficient

1.116   Context-sensitive half-time:

☐   A   Describes the time necessary for the plasma drug concentration to halve after the cessation of a continuous infusion designed to maintain a constant plasma concentration

☐   B   Bears a constant relationship to the drug elimination half-time

☐   C   Is high if the conductance ratio is high

☐   D   Of propofol after 2 hours is of the order of 20 minutes

☐   E   Of remifentanil is relatively constant

1.115 Answers:

- A True
- B False
- C False
- D True
- E False

A high inspired concentration leads to a rapid rise in P_A, as does an increase in alveolar ventilation. A large FRC will in effect dilute the inhaled anaesthetic agent and lead to a lower P_A. A high cardiac output maintains a constant gradient for diffusion of the anaesthetic agent and therefore the P_A rises more slowly. A high blood : gas partition coefficient means that the agent has a high solubility and therefore diffuses easily, so reducing P_A. The oil: gas partition coefficient affects the potency and therefore the minimum alveolar concentration (MAC) of the agent.

1.116 Answers:

- A True
- B False
- C True
- D True
- E True

The context-sensitive half-time of a drug may differ markedly from the elimination half-life. The elimination half-life does not take into account the pharmacokinetics of a multi-compartmental model. The conductance ratio describes the effect of elimination and distribution on the reduction of drug from the central compartment, ie plasma. A high conductance ratio signifies that a large amount of drug returns from the peripheral compartments into the plasma after cessation of drug. A low conductance ratio signifies that the redistribution of drug from the peripheral compartments into plasma is slow and so the drug is rapidly metabolised and the plasma level is kept low/insignificant.

The context-sensitive half-time of remifentanil is relatively constant at approximately 3 minutes as it is rapidly metabolised by plasma and tissue esterases.

1.117   The following drugs have a volume of distribution greater than 4 l/kg:

☐ A   Thiopental

☐ B   Atracurium

☐ C   Digoxin

☐ D   Flecainide

☐ E   Midazolam

1.118   The following are correct statements regarding drug response:

☐ A   Hyperreactivity describes an allergic response to a drug

☐ B   Tolerance to a drug that develops acutely is known as tachyphylaxis

☐ C   Cellular tolerance is the most important factor in the development of opioid tolerance

☐ D   The combination of two volatile anaesthetic agents would have a synergistic effect

☐ E   Desensitisation can occur secondary to a structural change in receptor morphology

1.117 Answers:

- A False
- B False
- C True
- D True
- E False

Volume of distribution of a drug is altered by plasma and tissue protein binding, the distribution of the drug to the tissues (ie lipid solubility and molecular size) and their blood flow. Drugs that have a large volume of distribution, ie >4 l/kg, include propofol, fentanyl, flecainide and digoxin (secondary to its affinity to bind to cardiac tissue). Thiopental has a V_d of 2.5 l/kg. Atracurium has a V_d of 0.15 l/kg. Midazolam has a V_d of 1.5 l/kg.

1.118 Answers:

- A False
- B True
- C True
- D False
- E True

Hyperreactivity is said to occur when unusually small doses of drug produce the expected pharmacological effect. The commonest cause of tachyphylaxis is secondary to depletion of stores, a common example being the decreasing effect seen with repetitive use of ephedrine as norepinephrine stores are depleted. Neuronal adaptation or cellular tolerance is seen with opioids, barbiturates and alcohol. This reflects a reduction in sensitivity of receptors in the CNS because of either reduction in number or sensitivity. A synergistic effect is seen when two drugs cause a greater pharmacological response than that expected by simple addition of their individual responses. The effect of using two volatile agents is additive.

Desensitisation occurs over a long period because of either receptor loss or structural change.

Reference: Hysteresis in drug response. *Anaesthesia and Intensive Care Medicine* 2005; 6: 286–7.

1.119 The following drugs have active metabolites:

☐ A Etomidate

☐ B Pancuronium

☐ C Lithium

☐ D Ciprofloxacin

☐ E Gentamicin

1.120 The following are metabolised by plasma cholinesterases:

☐ A Suxamethonium

☐ B Mivacurium

☐ C Cisatracurium

☐ D Esmolol

☐ E Remifentanil

1.119 Answers:

- A False
- B True
- C False
- D True
- E False

Of the intravenous induction agents, ketamine and thiopental have active metabolites. Propofol and etomidate do not. Of the muscle relaxants, pancuronium and vecuronium have active metabolites whereas atracurium (metabolite being laudanosine), cisatracurium, mivacurium and rocuronium (predominantly excreted unchanged) do not have active metabolites. Ciprofloxacin metabolites are active. A large range of antibiotics, including the aminoglycosides, is excreted unchanged and therefore they have no metabolites. Lithium is excreted unchanged by the kidneys.

1.120 Answers:

- A True
- B True
- C False
- D False
- E True

Cisatracurium, unlike atracurium, is not directly metabolised by plasma esterases. It undergoes Hofmann degradation. Its metabolites are then hydrolysed by non-specific plasma esterases. Esmolol is metabolised by red cell esterases. Remifentanil is metabolised by non-specific plasma and tissue cholinesterase.

1.121 Tachyphylaxis occurs with the following drugs:

☐ A Ephedrine

☐ B Morphine

☐ C Sodium nitroprusside

☐ D Trimetaphan

☐ E Esmolol

1.122 The following drugs preferentially act at α_2-adrenoreceptors:

☐ A Clonidine

☐ B Yohimbine

☐ C Phenoxybenzamine

☐ D Metaraminol

☐ E Prazosin

1.121 Answers:

- A True
- B False
- C True
- D True
- E False

Tachyphylaxis is the rapid reduction of effect after short-term administration of a drug. It is commonly secondary to depletion of neurotransmitters, eg norepinephrine in the case of ephedrine.

1.122 Answers:

- A True
- B True
- C False
- D False
- E False

Clonidine is a partial agonist at the α_2-receptor ($\alpha_2 : \alpha_1 = 200 : 1$), causing analgesia, sedation and hypotension. Prazosin is a highly selective postsynaptic α_1-blocker, causing hypotension and bladder sphincter relaxation. Phenoxybenzamine is a long-acting non-selective α-blocker with a higher affinity for the α_1- than the α_2-receptor. Metaraminol is a synthetic amine that is an α_1-agonist with some β-adrenoceptor activity. Yohimbine is a selective α_2-blocker that was used in the treatment of impotence.

1.123 Clonidine:

- ☐ A Reduces MAC
- ☐ B When administered with opioids, it potentiates their respiratory depressant effect
- ☐ C Can be administered to stop shivering
- ☐ D Causes a more profound reduction in diastolic compared with systolic blood pressure
- ☐ E Has an oral bioavailability of nearly 100%

1.124 Regarding prazosin:

- ☐ A It is a postsynaptic α_2-antagonist
- ☐ B It is used to relieve vasospasm in the Raynaud phenomenon
- ☐ C It should be stopped when screening urine for vanillyl-mandelic acid
- ☐ D It causes an increase in renin release
- ☐ E It can exaggerate the hypotension seen during epidural anaesthesia

1.123 Answers:

- A True
- B False
- C True
- D False
- E True

Clonidine is a centrally acting partial α_2-agonist. Acting centrally it causes a reduction in sympathetic outflow. MAC appears to be reduced by up to 50%. Clonidine does not cause or potentiate the respiratory depression seen with opioids. It is used to stop shivering at doses of 75 µg. This may be due to its ability to inhibit central thermoregulatory control. Its cardiovascular effect is more profound on systolic rather than diastolic pressures. It has the desirable effect of decreasing systemic blood pressure without paralysis of compensatory homoeostatic mechanisms. It has excellent oral bioavailability, reaching its maximum plasma level within 90 minutes. It is minimally protein bound (20%) and has a volume of distribution of 2 l/kg.

1.124 Answers:

- A False
- B True
- C True
- D False
- E True

Prazosin is a selective postsynaptic α_1-adrenergic receptor antagonist. It causes vasodilatation of both arteries and veins, but has greater affinity for venous α-receptors. This causes it to have postural hypotensive effects similar to GTN. It does not cause reflex tachycardia or release of renin. This is because α_2-receptors are unaffected and they inhibit the release of renin. Due to the α_1-blockade caused by prazosin, the usual compensatory vasoconstriction mechanism is lost. Therefore, hypotension with epidurals may be exaggerated, as the vessels not affected by the epidural are unable to vasoconstrict. Prazosin must be stopped before screening for urinary catecholamine metabolites, as it can yield a false-positive result.

1.125 Activated charcoal:

- ☐ A Is most effective if used within the first hour of ingestion
- ☐ B Has its principal mode of action in the lower gastrointestinal tract
- ☐ C Before use is activated using oxidising gas
- ☐ D Is effective in chelating lithium
- ☐ E Should be used as first-line treatment of early methanol poisoning

1.125 Answers:

- A True
- B False
- C True
- D False
- E False

Activated charcoal is a fine, black, odourless and tasteless powder made from wood or other materials that have been exposed to very high temperatures in an airless environment. It is then activated to increase its ability to adsorb various substances, by reheating with oxidising gas or other chemicals, so breaking it into a very fine powder. Activated charcoal is pure carbon specially processed to make it highly adsorbent of particles and gases. It is most effective when given within the first hour of ingestion and when only small amounts have been ingested. Its principal site of action is gastric and in the small intestine. Dosage is 50–100 g/4 hours or 25 g/2 hours. It is effective for chelating barbiturates and tricyclic antidepressants but is ineffective for lithium, ethanol and methanol poisoning.

Reference: www.toxbase.org

1.126 The following are correctly paired with their appropriate chelating agent:

☐ A Dicobalt and lead poisoning

☐ B Ferrihaemate and iron poisoning

☐ C Activated charcoal and amitriptyline

☐ D Thiocyanate and cyanide

☐ E Dimercaprol and gold

1.126 Answers:

- A False
- B False
- C True
- D False
- E True

A chelating agent binds a toxic substance and prevents tissue damage. Thiocyanate is formed in the liver and kidneys, when a cyanide ion combines with a sulphydryl group. Sodium thiosulphate provides more sulphydryl groups to facilitate the conversion of cyanide ions to thiocyanate. Ferrihaemate is a nephrotoxic breakdown product of myoglobin in acidic conditions.

Chelating agent	Chelates
Desferrioxamine	Iron, aluminium
Dimercaprol	Arsenic, bismuth, mercury, gold
Sodium calcium edetate	Lead, copper, radioactive metals
Penicillamine	Copper, lead, gold, mercury, zinc
Dicobalt	Cyanide

1.127   The following is true regarding the vitamin K-dependent clotting factors:

☐   A   The half-life of factor II is by far the longest

☐   B   These factors include factor XI

☐   C   Oestrogen increases their production.

☐   D   Carbamazepine reduces the effect of warfarin on them

☐   E   After receiving warfarin factor VII is the first to become depleted

1.128   The following may increase the effect of warfarin:

☐   A   Amiodarone

☐   B   D-Thyroxine

☐   C   Acute illness

☐   D   Broad-spectrum antibiotics

☐   E   Cholestyramine

1.127   Answers:

- A   True
- B   False
- C   True
- D   True
- E   True

Factors II, VII, IX and X are the vitamin K-dependent clotting factors. Their half-lives are 60 hours, 6 hours, 24 hours and 40 hours respectively. Therefore, following warfarin treatment factor VII, with the shortest half-life, is depleted first. Oestrogens increase their production. Carbamazepine reduces the effect of warfarin and therefore reduces the depletion of vitamin K-dependent clotting factors.

Reference: Anticoagulants and the perioperative period. *Continuing Education in Anaesthesia, Critical Care and Pain* 2006; 6(4): 156–9.

1.128   Answers:

- A   True
- B   True
- C   True
- D   True
- E   True

The effects of warfarin can be potentiated by displacing warfarin from its protein binding or by decreasing vitamin K absorption.

Amiodarone displaces warfarin from its binding sites and therefore increases the free fraction and therefore effect. D-Thyroxine increases the potency of warfarin by increasing hepatic receptor sites, as does quinidine. Acute illness reduces vitamin K absorption. Broad-spectrum antibiotics reduce the level of gut bacteria required for vitamin K absorption. Cholestyramine decreases vitamin K absorption.

Reference: Anticoagulants and the perioperative period. *Continuing Education in Anaesthesia, Critical Care and Pain* 2006; 6(4): 156–9.

1.129   Drug effect on platelets:

☐   A   Aspirin inhibits prostaglandin production

☐   B   Selective cyclo-oxygenase (COX)-2 antagonists cause
significant platelet dysfunction

☐   C   Dipyridamole inhibits platelet metabolism of adenosine.

☐   D   Clopidogrel blocks the ADP-induced platelet activation
pathway

☐   E   Platelet glycoprotein IIb/IIIa antagonists also reduce thrombin
concentration

1.129   Answers:

- A   True
- B   False
- C   True
- D   True
- E   True

Aspirin inhibits both prostaglandin and thromboxane production. Selective COX-2 antagonists do not cause significant platelet dysfunction. Dipyridamole may have a number of mechanisms of action, including the one in option C. It may also have its effects via prostacyclin. It potentiates its effect by being a phosphodiesterase inhibitor and also by directly stimulating the release of prostacyclin by the endothelium.

Reference: Anticoagulants and the perioperative period. *Continuing Education in Anaesthesia, Critical Care and Pain* 2006; 6(4): 156–9.

CLINICAL

MCQs

Indicate your answers with a tick or cross in the boxes provided.

1.130 Basic calculations in children: the following are appropriate doses for children during resuscitation:

☐ A Amiodarone 5 μg/kg

☐ B 5 ml/kg 10% dextrose for a hypoglycaemic child

☐ C 2 J/kg for initial DC cardioversion of ventricular fibrillation

☐ D 0.1 mg/kg epinephrine for resuscitation of asystole

☐ E 20 ml/kg fluid bolus for hypovolaemia

1.131 The following are true of calculations for children:

☐ A The Broselow tape relates height to weight

☐ B The estimated weight of a term newborn is 2 kg

☐ C The estimated systolic blood pressure of a child can be derived from the following equation 80 + (age in years × 4)

☐ D The appropriate size cannula for a cricothyroidotomy in an infant would be 18 gauge

☐ E Approximate weight of a child aged 1–10 years can be calculate by the equation (age in years + 4) × 2

1.130 Answers:

- A False
- B True
- C False
- D False
- E True

The following doses are correct for resuscitation of a child:

- epinephrine 0.1 ml/kg of 1:10 000, which is equivalent to 10 µg/kg
- amiodarone 5 mg/kg
- 5 ml/kg 10% dextrose
- fluid bolus of 20 ml/kg for resuscitation of hypovolaemia
- 4 J/kg for DC shock.

Reference: *Advance Paediatric Life Support Course Manual.* Fourth edition. (Updated January 2006)

1.131 Answers:

- A True
- B False
- C False
- D True
- E True

The Broselow tape was designed to estimate body weight, drug dosage and endotracheal tube size in paediatric emergencies, based on patient height. A study performed in 2002 (*British Journal of Anaesthesia* 2002; 88: 283–5) showed that it provided accurate estimation of body weight based on measured body length but it slightly underestimated body weight in all cases. In smaller children, <20 kg, this underestimate was negligible but was more pronounced in children >20 kg. Tracheal tube size met clinical needs better than age-based estimates.

The estimated weight of a newborn is 3.5 kg at term. Systolic blood pressure can be calculated using 80 + (age × 2). The cannula sizes recommended by APLS (Advanced Paediatric Life Support) for cricothyroidotomy are 18 gauge in an infant and 14 gauge for a child.

Reference: *Advance Paediatric Life Support course manual* - The practical approach. Fourth edition (Updated January 2006); *British Journal of Anaesthesia* 2002; 88(2): 283–5.

1.132   When diagnosing malignant hyperthermia (MH):

☐   A   A negative family history precludes the diagnosis

☐   B   Having identified a MH patient, the family members can be reassured that they are not MH susceptible if they have a normal DNA test

☐   C   A rise in postoperative temperature with no preceding tachycardia or increased CO_2 production could be MH

☐   D   It can occur after cessation of the trigger

☐   E   All patients with central core disease should be suspected of being potential MH sufferers

1.132 Answers:

- A False
- B False
- C False
- D False
- E True

The inheritance of MH was initially thought to be in an autosomal dominant fashion. This is now known not to be the case. There are to date 15 clinically relevant gene mutations for the ryanodine receptor protein (RYR)1. There are also several other genetic loci not associated with RYR1 that have been linked with MH in some families. In other families, no genetic abnormality has been found. Once an abnormal gene has been identified in one family member, other family members can be DNA tested. If the abnormal gene is found they are known to be MH patients. However, a normal DNA test does not exclude MH susceptibility (ie false-negative result) and therefore the family member should go on to have muscle biopsy and contracture testing.

The exclusion of MH based on intraoperative events is dependent of the calibre of the perioperative records. A late rise in temperature without preceding tachycardia and increased CO_2 production is not MH. MH cannot commence once the trigger has been removed. Central core disease is an inherited disorder causing peripheral muscle weakness that is associated with MH.

Reference: Malignant hyperthermia. *British Journal of Anaesthesia CEPD Reviews* 2003; 3(1): 5–9.

1.133 Regarding malignant hyperpyrexia:

☐ A Vigorous cooling is always beneficial

☐ B Dantrolene must be mixed in dextrose

☐ C Myoglobinuria occurs before a rise in creatine kinase (CK)

☐ D Low concentrations of volatile anaesthesia may give rise to a more insidious onset

☐ E An alkaline diuresis may reduce post MH renal failure

1.133   Answers:

- A   False
- B   False
- C   True
- D   True
- E   True

MH is a condition of uncontrolled muscular contraction owing to a defect in intracellular calcium homoeostasis. This leads to persistent muscle contraction with its accompanying metabolic sequelae, including tachycardia, increased CO_2 production, acidosis, hyperthermia and rhabdomyolysis.

Dantrolene prevents calcium release from the sarcoplasmic reticulum, so reducing the reaction. It is presented as a powder with mannitol and sodium hydroxide. It is reconstituted in 60 ml water per 20 mg vial.

Myoglobinuria is apparent before CK increases, the peak CK rise being approximately 24 hours after the insult. One causative agent of renal failure in rhabdomyolysis is ferrihaemate, a nephrotoxic breakdown product in acidic conditions. Alkalinisation of urine promotes its excretion.

Vigorous cooling can lead to severe peripheral vasoconstriction that can actually cause a rise in core temperature.

Reference: Malignant hyperthermia. *British Journal of Anaesthesia CEPD Reviews* 2003; 3(1): 5–9.

1.134 Pre-eclampsia:

☐ A Occurs in the first trimester

☐ B Is diagnosed as severe if the patient presents with pulmonary oedema

☐ C Is associated with uric acid concentrations of >360 µmol/l

☐ D Is associated with a decrease in thromboxane production

☐ E Associated with HELLP syndrome occurs post partum in 50% of cases

1.134 Answers:

- A False
- B True
- C True
- D False
- E False

Pre-eclampsia can be diagnosed in pregnancy after 20 weeks. It classically presents as a triad of hypertension, proteinuria and oedema. It is defined as mild, moderate or severe. Severe pre-eclampsia is defined as any one of the following: severe hypertension (SBP > 160 mmHg, DBP > 110 mmHg); proteinuria > 5 g/24 h; oliguria < 400 ml/24 h; cerebral irritation; epigastric or right upper quadrant pain; pulmonary oedema.

The precise aetiology of pre-eclampsia is unknown. Placental insufficiency causing ischaemia results in the release of vasoactive substances that cause a multi-system disorder. Thromboxane production increases and prostacyclin concentration decreases, which cause platelet dysfunction and vasoconstriction. **HELLP** syndrome – **h**aemolysis, **e**levated **l**iver enzymes and **l**ow **p**latelets – occurs with severe pre-eclampsia in up to 50% of cases. Around 20% of cases occur post partum.

Reference: Diagnosis and management of pre-eclampsia. *British Journal of Anaesthesia CEPD Reviews* 2003; 2(2): 38–42.

1.135 When managing severe pre-eclampsia:

☐ A CVP monitoring is valuable as it gives a good correlation with left atrial pressure

☐ B Before loading with magnesium, fluid is required for volume expansion

☐ C A mean BP of less than 80 mmHg is ideal

☐ D The severity of hypertension correlates well with the incidence of progression to eclampsia

☐ E Magnesium dose is calculated according to serum concentration

1.135 Answers:

- A False
- B True
- C False
- D False
- E False

Central venous pressure (CVP) monitoring can be used to gauge fluid requirement; however, it is known to be a poor correlator with left atrial pressure, particularly in severe pre-eclampsia.

The vasodilatory effect of magnesium is counteracted by cautious fluid administration. This is particularly important antenatally to maintain adequate placental perfusion. A profound reduction in blood pressure should be avoided as this compromises placental circulation. Aim for mean blood pressure of 100–140 mmHg. Hypertension severity correlates poorly with development of eclampsia. Magnesium levels are not routinely titrated to serum values. Respiratory rate, tendon reflexes and urine output are closely monitored. Magnesium is renally excreted. If the patient is anuric, magnesium therapy is reduced and levels may be useful.

Reference: Diagnosis and management of pre-eclampsia. *British Journal of Anaesthesia CEPD Reviews* 2003; 2(2): 38–42.

1.136 Regarding HIV infection and treatment:

☐ A Zidovudine inhibits the synthesis of DNA by reverse
          transcriptase

☐ B Non-nucleoside reverse transcriptase inhibitors bind to reverse
          transcriptase and inhibit enzyme activity

☐ C Protease inhibitors decrease the effect of opiates

☐ D The average risk of transmission of HIV following muco-
          cutaneous contact is 10 times less than following needle-stick
          injury

☐ E Myocarditis is common in HIV sufferers

1.136 Answers:

- A True
- B True
- C False
- D True
- E True

Treatment for HIV is broadly split into three groups. Nucleoside analogue reverse transcriptase inhibitors (NRTIs), eg zidovudine, act as a false nucleotide so preventing the production of DNA from viral RNA. Non-nucleoside reverse transcriptase inhibitors (NNRTIs) bind to reverse transcriptase preventing enzyme activity. Protease inhibitors (PIs) prevent production of active viral proteins. HAART or highly active antiretroviral therapy consists of two NRTIs and either a PI or an NNRTI. PIs inhibit the metabolism of opioids and benzodiazepines.

The average risk of transmission after a needle stick injury is 0.3% compared with mucocutaneous contact when it is 0.03%.

Up to 50% of HIV sufferers will have an abnormal ECG. Myocarditis is common secondary to drugs, lymphoma, opportunistic infection or the disease itself.

Reference: Anaesthesia and critical care for patients with HIV infection. *Continuing Education in Anaesthesia, Critical Care and Pain* 2005; 5(5): 153–6.

1.137 Anaesthesia for non-obstetric surgery during pregnancy:

- ☐ A Teratogenicity risk to the fetus is greatest during the first 14 days of gestation
- ☐ B Non-steroidal anti-inflammatory drugs are safe to use for pain relief
- ☐ C Ideally, surgery should be performed before commencement of the second trimester
- ☐ D Antacid prophylaxis is recommended from the beginning of the second trimester
- ☐ E MAC (minimum alveolar concentration) is increased in pregnancy

1.138 After intra-arterial injection of thiopental, the following may be of benefit:

- ☐ A Intra-arterial papaverine
- ☐ B Intravenous guanethidine
- ☐ C Stellate ganglion block
- ☐ D Brachial plexus block
- ☐ E Intra-arterial procaine

1.137 Answers:

- A False
- B False
- C False
- D True
- E False

Teratogenicity is greatest between days 15 and 56 of gestation. If possible surgery is postponed until the second trimester to reduce the risk of teratogenicity and miscarriage. Non-steroidal anti-inflammatory drugs are contraindicated in pregnancy secondary to the risk of closure of the fetal ductus arteriosus. MAC decreases in pregnancy from as early as 8 weeks' gestation. Also, remember the risk of uterine atony with volatile anaesthesia.

Reference: Anaesthesia for non-obstetrical surgery during pregnancy. *Continuing Education in Anaesthesia, Critical Care and Pain* 2006; 6(2): 83–85.

1.138 Answers:

- A True
- B True
- C True
- D True
- E True

Intra-arterial injection of thiopental causes intense pain. The thiopental crystallises in arterioles and capillaries and there is local release of norepinephrine causing vasospasm. Treatment is aimed at pain reduction and counteracting the vasospasm.

After intra-arterial injection, the cannula should be left in situ; 5 ml 0.5% procaine (local anaesthetic for analgesia) and 40 mg papaverine (vasodilator) should be injected. Other treatment options include sympathetic blockade either with a stellate ganglion or brachial plexus block or with intravenous guanethidine.

1.139 The following is true of the Vaughan–Williams classification of anti-arrhythmic drugs:

☐ A Ibutilide is a class III anti-arrhythmic

☐ B All β-blockers are class II anti-arrhythmics

☐ C Calcium channel blockers are class IV

☐ D Class III drugs shorten repolarisation

☐ E Class IC drugs prolong repolarisation

1.139 Answers:

- A True
- B False
- C True
- D False
- E False

Class IA	Prolong repolarisation	Quinidine, procainamide, disopyramide
Class IB	Shorten repolarisation	Lidocaine, mexiletine, phenytoin, tocainide
Class IC	Little effect on repolarisation	Encainide, flecainide, propafenone
Class II	β-Adrenergic blockade	Propranolol, esmolol, acebutolol, L-sotalol
Class III	Prolonged repolarisation (potassium channel blockade; other)	Amiodarone, bretylium, D- or L-sotalol, ibutilide, dofetilide
Class IV	Calcium channel blockade	Verapamil, diltiazem, bepridil

- The β-blocker sotalol is in both classes II and III.
- Ibutilide and dofetilide are examples of class III drugs that are recommended for first-line therapy in patients with atrial fibrillation (AF) of <7 days' duration, as are flecainide and propafenone.

  Reference: ACC/AHA/ESC Guidelines for the management of patients with atrial fibrillation: executive summary. *Circulation* 2001; 104: 2118–50.

1.140 Amiodarone in AF:

☐ A Provides swift rate control secondary to its class III effect

☐ B Has a toxicity that is predominantly dose dependent

☐ C Can be changed for flecainide as a reasonable alternative in patients with ischaemic heart disease

☐ D Is currently recommended as first choice for pharmacological cardioversion of less than 7 days' duration

☐ E Can offer additional benefit when given intravenously to patients who are fully loaded with oral amiodarone therapy

1.140 Answers:

- A False
- B True
- C False
- D False
- E True

The swift rate control of amiodarone in AF is secondary to its β-blockade and calcium channel-blocking effect. Its anti-arrhythmic effects start 8–24 hours later.

Current guidelines (ACC/AHA/ESC Guidelines for the management of patients with atrial fibrillation: executive summary. *Circulation* 2001; 104: 2118–50) recommend the use of propafenone, flecainide, ibutilide and dofetilide as first-line therapy for AF of less than 7 days' duration.

Both intravenous and oral amiodarone may have different electrophysiological properties and so intravenous preparations may offer additional benefit to patients already on loaded oral therapy.

Reference: Atrial fibrillation. *Continuing Education in Anaesthesia, Critical Care and Pain* 6(6): 219–24.

1.141 Regarding elective DC cardioversion in AF:

☐ A Success is increased with anterior–posterior positioning of paddles compared with anterior–lateral positioning

☐ B Following cardioversion, a rise in cardiac troponins signifies cardiac damage

☐ C When using a monophasic defibrillator, the initial energy selected is 200 J.

☐ D It should be preceded by anticoagulation if the patient has been in AF for over 24 hours

☐ E It is contraindicated in patients with internal defibrillators

1.141 Answers:

- A True
- B False
- C True
- D False
- E False

When using monophasic defibrillators, an initial energy of 200 J is recommended. With further direct currents set at 200, 300 then 360 J.

Following cardioversion, a transient rise in ST segments and cardiac troponins can occur even without cardiac damage.

Anticoagulation should be achieved if the patient has been in AF for longer than 48 hours and should be continued for 3–4 weeks following successful cardioversion. Chronic AF is associated with a 3–7% annual risk of CVA (cerebrovascular accident). DC cardioversion of AF is not contraindicated by internal defibrillators or pacemakers; however, they should be interrogated before and after cardioversion. The paddle position is placed as far from the device as possible, preferably anterior–posterior.

Reference: Atrial fibrillation. Continuing education in anaesthesia, critical care and pain. *British Journal of Anaesthesia* 6(6): 219–24.

1.142 With regard to preoperative fasting:

☐ A Gastric emptying of liquid is an exponential process

☐ B 95% of ingested clear fluid is emptied from the stomach within 1 hour

☐ C Obesity delays gastric emptying

☐ D Residual gastric volumes are smaller with prolonged fasting

☐ E Regurgitation is common in the first 6 months of life

1.142 Answers:

- A True
- B True
- C False
- D False
- E True

Obesity does not delay gastric emptying. It does, however, increase the risk of hiatus hernia and other associated pathologies. Studies show that longer starvation periods cause an increase in residual gastric volume when compared with shorter times.

In the first 6 months of life, the intragastric pressure is high as the stomach is small and compressed by other intra-abdominal organs.

The accepted guidelines for starvation:

- 2 hours   water and clear fluids
- 4 hours   breast milk
- 6 hours   drinks with milk, food and sweets.

See Royal College of Nursing, *Recommendations for Preoperative Fasting* 2005.

Reference: Pre-operative fasting. *Continuing Education in Anaesthesia, Critical Care and Pain* 2006; 6(6): 215–18.

1.143 Regarding blood and blood transfusion:

☐ A A massive blood transfusion is defined as more than 6 units of blood within 8 hours

☐ B Fresh frozen plasma (FFP) and platelet additive solutions contain significant amounts of citrate compared with red blood cell (RBC) concentrates

☐ C Hyperkalaemia is common in massive transfusion

☐ D Naturally occurring anti-A antibody in B blood groups is of IgM class

☐ E Antibodies resulting from transplacental passage are of IgM class

1.143 Answers:

- A False
- B True
- C False
- D True
- E False

Massive transfusion is defined as the replacement of a patient's total blood volume in less than 24 hours. Hyperkalaemia after a massive transfusion is uncommon unless the patient is acidotic and hypothermic. This is because the RBC membrane's NA^+/K^+ pumping mechanism is quickly re-established, which clears the potassium load of the transfused blood. Hypocalcaemia can occur because of the chelating effect of citrate, which is in higher concentrations in FFP and platelets. Transplacentally acquired antibodies are IgG.

Reference: Complications of blood transfusion. *Continuing Education in Anaesthesia, Critical Care and Pain* 2006; 6(6): 225–9.

1.144 TRALI (transfusion-related acute lung injury):

- ☐ A Occurs within 6 hours of a blood transfusion
- ☐ B Is antibody mediated in approximately 90% of cases
- ☐ C Is caused by activation of neutrophil granulocyte cells
- ☐ D In non-antibody-mediated cases, has a lower mortality
- ☐ E Is more commonly caused by FFP than RBC products

1.144 Answers:

- A True
- B False
- C True
- D True
- E True

TRALI causes acute respiratory distress within 6 hours of a blood transfusion. There are two mechanisms: immune (or antibody mediated in 60% of cases) and non-immune mediated. Immune mediated TRALI is caused by leukocyte antibodies in the donor blood reacting with recipient human leukocyte antigens and human neutrophil alloantigens. Non-immune mediated TRALI is not caused by leukocytes but by reactive lipid products released from donor blood cell membranes. The common final pathway is the activation of neutrophil granulocyte cells that migrate to the lungs and become trapped. Free radicals and proteolytic enzymes are released causing a capillary leak and pulmonary oedema. FFP and platelets contain more plasma and therefore are more likely to cause TRALI.

Reference: Complications of blood transfusion. *Continuing Education in Anaesthesia, Critical Care and Pain* 2006; 6(6): 225–9.

1.145 Basic life support (BLS) in adults (updated guidelines December 2005):

☐ A On confirmation of cardiac arrest, two effective breaths should be administered

☐ B Chest compression should be commenced at a rate of 100 per minute

☐ C The chest compression to breath ratio is 30 : 2

☐ D Chest compression-only cardiopulmonary resuscitation (CPR) is effective for a limited period only

☐ E Transmission of HIV during CPR has occurred

1.145   Answers:

- A False
- B True
- C True
- D True
- E False

Current teaching now enforces immediate administration of chest compressions before effective breath administration. This is to reduce the pause before compressions. Chest compression-only CPR has been highlighted as there is a reluctance to perform mouth-to-mouth ventilation. Chest compression-only CPR is only effective for approximately 5 minutes. There have been no documented cases of HIV transmission during CPR administration.

Reference: *Advanced Life Support.* 5th edn. Resuscitation Council (UK) April 2006.

1.146   Regarding cardiac arrest in adults:

☐ A   It is the leading cause of death in European adults

☐ B   Successful resuscitation is likely if the original ECG is asystolic

☐ C   The delay from collapse to delivery of the first shock decreases the chance of survival from ventricular fibrillation (VF) by 10% per minute

☐ D   BLS helps maintain a shockable rhythm for deterioration to asystole

☐ E   Current guidelines for treatment of VF recommend the delivery of a single shock, then returning to CPR

1.147   The following is correct regarding the management of VF:

☐ A   After a single shock, CPR is continued for 2 minutes before a rhythm check

☐ B   All monophasic shocks for defibrillation should be at 360 J

☐ C   Epinephrine should be administered if VF/VT persists after the second defibrillation

☐ D   Amiodarone should be given after two unsuccessful defibrillations

☐ E   Fine VF should be defibrillated immediately

Clinical MCQs

1.146 Answers:

- A True
- B False
- C True
- D True
- E True

  Asystole or PEA (pulseless electrical activity) is associated with an extremely poor survival outcome. BLS is not definitive treatment for a shockable rhythm but helps to maintain a shockable rhythm until such time as defibrillation is available.

  Reference: *Advanced Life Support*. 5th edn. Resuscitation Council (UK) April 2006.

1.147 Answers:

- A True
- B True
- C True
- D False
- E False

  Recommended initial energy for a biphasic defibrillator is 150–200 J, with second and subsequent shocks at 150–360 J. Amiodarone should be given if VF/VT (VT = ventricular tachycardia) persists after a third shock. The chance of successfully shocking fine VF is very unlikely. Good quality CPR may improve the amplitude and frequency of VF and so improve the likelihood of successful defibrillation. Repeated delivery of shocks increases myocardial injury.

  Reference: *Advanced Life Support*. 5th edn. Resuscitation Council (UK) April 2006.

1.148 The following are true regarding ALS guidelines:

    ☐ A Precordial thump is delivered over the apex

    ☐ B Single shock protocol compared with three stacked shocks decreases the CPR-free period and improves chances of survival

    ☐ C The first shock efficacy of a biphasic waveform is >90%

    ☐ D Asystolic rhythm should be reassessed every 2 minutes

    ☐ E During defibrillation oxygen masks should be held at least 1 metre away from the patient's chest

1.149 Drugs used in during cardiac arrest:

    ☐ A Epinephrine should be given every cycle

    ☐ B Lidocaine may be given for refractory VF at a dose of 2 mg/kg

    ☐ C If the rhythm is slow PEA (<60 beats/min) atropine 3 mg should be administered

    ☐ D Vasopressin is the new vasopressor of choice in VF arrest

    ☐ E 10 ml 10% calcium chloride contains less Ca^{2+} than 10 ml 10% calcium gluconate

1.148 Answers:

- A False
- B True
- C True
- D True
- E True

A precordial thump should be delivered only after a witnessed cardiac arrest. A sharp impact should be administered to the lower half of the sternum from a height of approximately 20 cm. It is much more likely to convert a VT to sinus rhythm than VF. In all reported successful cases, the precordial thump was given within the first 10 seconds.

Reference: *Advanced Life Support*. 5th edn. Resuscitation Council (UK) April 2006.

1.149 Answers:

- A False
- B False
- C True
- D False
- E False

A dose of 1 mg epinephrine should be administered every 3–5 minutes, not necessarily every cycle if on the shockable side of the algorithm. If amiodarone is not available, lidocaine 1 mg/kg can be used as an alternative. Vasopressin shows no statistically significant difference in the rate of death before hospital discharge when compared with epinephrine; 10 ml 10% calcium chloride contains 6.8 mmol Ca^{2+} and 10 ml 10% calcium gluconate contains 2.2 mmol Ca^{2+}.

Reference: *Advanced Lfe Support*. 5th edn. Resuscitation Council (UK) April 2006.

1.150 Paediatric resuscitation:

☐ A An infant is defined as <1 year old

☐ B Standard automated external defibrillators (AEDs) can be safely used in children <8 years old

☐ C Upon confirmation of no breath two rescue breaths should be given

☐ D Two-person resuscitation utilises a ratio of 15 : 2 chest compressions to breaths

☐ E Assistance should be sought after 1 minute of unsuccessful CPR

1.150 Answers:

- A True
- B False
- C False
- D True
- E True

Infants are defined as <1 year old. A child is between 1 year and puberty. Standard AEDs can safely be used in children over the age of 8 years. Purpose-made paediatric pads or programmes that attenuate the energy output of an AED are recommended for children under 8 years. Current practice supports the administration of five rescue breaths after confirmation of absent respiration. Only in cases of a child with a witnessed sudden collapse should a rescuer not perform 1 minute CPR before calling for help.

Reference: *Advanced Paediatric Life Support.* 4th edn. (updated January 2006).

CORE TEXT REFERENCES

Peck TE, Williams M. and Hill SA. *Pharmacology for Anaesthesia and Intensive Care*. 2nd edn. G.M.M. 2003.

Stoelting RK and Hillier SC. *Pharmacology and Physiology in Anaesthetic Practice*. 4th edn. Lippincott Williams and Wilkins 2005.

Yentis SM, Hirsch NP and Smith GB. *Anaesthesia and Intensive Care A–Z. An encyclopedia of principles and practice*. 3rd edn. Butterworth Heinemann 2004.

INDEX

Locators in bold refer to book number, those in normal type refer to question number.

Index

Index

Index